HANDLING HARD STUFF (LIKE A #BOSS)

HOW TO NAVIGATE THE HARD PARTS OF LIFE WITH PURPOSE

COURTNEY ST CROIX, SHARANA ALI,
& THE CO-AUTHOR TEAM

Ali Martin | Ashleigh Stephens | Chantal Carruthers
Chloe-Jean Summers | Danielle Lehmkuhl | Dr. Mandy Lee
Jenna Peters | ML | Michelle Pfile | Nazia Shahrin
Nicole Bell | Peg Cleland | Taahirah Issany | Vicki Spindloe

leadher
PUBLISHING

HANDLING HARD STUFF (LIKE A #BOSS)

How To Navigate the Hard Parts of Life With Purpose

2022 LeadHer Publishing

Cover Design - Michelle Fairbanks / Fresh Design
Editing - Donna Zuniga and Megan Baker Jackson
Interior Design - Christina Williams
ISBN -978-1-990352-10-2
Book Cover, Typesetting, and Layout Design

For more information, visit www.lead-her.com
instagram.com/leadherpublishing
or email admin@lead-her.com

CONTENTS

Foreword: Courtney St Croix 7

Introduction: Sharana Ali 13

Chapter 1: Ali Martin 19

Chapter 2: Ashleigh Stephens 33

Chapter 3: Chantal Carruthers 51

Chapter 4: Chloe Jean Summers 65

Chapter 5: Danielle Lehmkuhl 79

Chapter 6: Dr. Mandy Lee 97

Chapter 7: Jenna Peters 111

Chapter 8: M.L. 125

Chapter 9: Michelle Pfile 135

Chapter 10: Nazia Shahrin 153

Chapter 11: Nicole Bell 165

Chapter 12: Peg Cleland 179

Chapter 13: Sharana Ali 191

Chapter 14: Taahirah Issany 201

Chapter 15: Vicki Spindloe 217

Foreword

COURTNEY ST CROIX

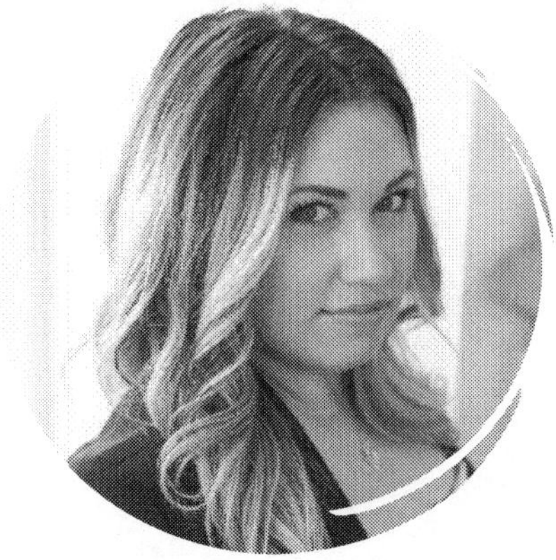

Photo: Leah Smith

@leadherpublishing
leadherpublishing.com

I was out for a walk sometime in Spring 2021 trying to break up the day so that my daughter and I got to see something other than the four walls of our house for at least a part of the day. At this time, we were told not to go anywhere other than for basic requirements like shopping for groceries, and... well, that was basically it. So we were at home a *lot*. My daughter was 5 at the time, and needless to say, the virtual school alternative was not going the smoothest in our household. It was really difficult trying to accomplish anything on my to-do list other than "wake up" and "have coffee." Having low productivity and accomplishment expectations was better for my mental health than the frustration that came with having high hopes and almost a guaranteed low rate of success—so getting out of the house was our accomplishment on this particular day.

While my daughter ran ahead on the park path, I popped my earbuds in and started listening to an audiobook. I remember feeling more overwhelmed than I had ever felt in my entire life up until that point. Everything was stressing me out. I felt over-stimulated by sounds and physical touch, and would regularly have loud outbursts that were not intentional but a product of circumstance. I had a sense of being "behind" that I still cannot really describe. I felt stuck. Frustrated. Annoyed. Guilty. Angry. Sad. Everything I felt on a regular basis was low vibrational and negative-toned, and all the days began to feel the same, blending into one another like neither had a beginning nor an end. I felt I was failing in nearly every area of my life, And I just needed a minute to disconnect. So my earbuds went in.

I was listening to *Think Like A Monk* by Jay Shetty (which is a book I highly recommend, by the way!). I am a person who is keenly aware of polarity and opposing viewpoints, so each time Jay explained something about your energy and your perspective being your choice, I felt a little slighted. Doesn't he know that things are *hard* right now? Doesn't he know it isn't all rainbows and sunshine in the world? Doesn't he know we're all struggling? Doesn't he know it isn't as easy as he says it is to just "turn things around?"

At the very moment I was contemplating his theories, he started to tell a story about trees. At first I wondered where he was going with this story, but I'm glad I paid attention. He said something (and I'm paraphrasing here, but I'd recommend this book for this takeaway alone!) about how there is a dendrology lab that studies the growth of trees, and in said lab they have many trees growing in a perfectly situated, temperature—and element-controlled indoor environment. The circumstances are perfect—so, as the theory went, the trees should be the healthiest and strongest damn trees on Earth. Their environment was perfectly controlled and simulated. They got everything they needed and were closely monitored as they grew. Things were going well, until one day, the scientists started noticing that at a certain level of growth, the trees would just simply fall over and die. At a certain height, they would give up. Quit. Topple. Or so it seemed.

After some head-scratching, testing, and more experiments, they finally realized what was missing inside their perfect, man-made, curated environment designed to help plants thrive...

Wind.

Logically, it would seem like wind is such a big stressor for trees—that keeping them from it should make them even better. They aren't at risk for breaking and falling and they would be able to stand taller and stronger.

But the wind is a necessary, normal, and healthy stressor for the life of a tree.
Wind helps trees build resiliency from the time they are tiny saplings to the time they are 30-year-old windswept pines.
Wind helps tree trunks get stronger under pressure.
Wind helps trees overcome challenges and thrive despite the circumstances.
Wind helps trees manage and prepare for future weather stressors.

By removing wind from the perfectly curated environment, the trees were so fragile that once they reached a certain height (and weight) the bottom of their trunks couldn't handle that amount of stress, and gravity would simply force them to the ground. They hadn't built any stress resiliency in order to successfully hold up their own weight.

I don't think I'll ever forget this story, and I use it regularly to help remind me that we need stress and pressure in order to survive and to thrive. Perfect conditions do not always equal perfect results. We need to learn how to manage alongside the wind in our lives, not run away from it. We can't hide from the wind; it's always there in some capacity. We can, however, learn how to manage it—if we pay attention—but we must understand that the wind challenges us with intention. It helps us dig in our roots and grow stronger, taller, bigger, and to rise up as the leaders of our own lives despite the adversity we face.

The human experience is a complex one, and I think you'd agree that we're all constantly inundated with our own forms of highs and lows; peaks and valleys that carry us through life. Some phases feel incredible, and others feel terrifying. We are essentially riding the waves of our lives, up and down, and I encourage you to consider giving value to the low points as much as you give value to the high ones.

Highs and lows.
Like waves in the ocean.
We are here to experience it all.

There is a saying that I've heard a lot as someone who spends a lot of time on the water:

"The sea is angry today."

The thing is, though, it's not actually the sea that's angry when the waves are crashing up against the shore.

It's the wind. The wind is angry. The wind is the underlying element that affects what the waves do. How the waves behave. We need the wind. We need the challenge. We need the pressure.

So we can rise above it.

Whatever you're going through in your life, I hope that you feel connected, seen, and heard through reading the stories of each author contributing to this anthology. We are all going through something, and we can all lean on each other in times of difficulty.

Stand tall in the face of a strong wind; you were designed to handle it.

You can do this.

Sending you strength and love,

Courtney St Croix

CEO, LeadHer Publishing

Introduction
SHARANA ALI

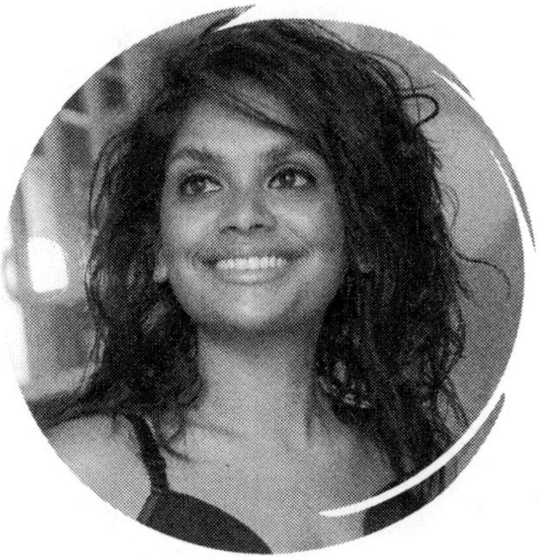

Instagram @BOSSTheSixEdition
Bossthesixedition@gmail.com

Like many, I grew up dreaming of the day I would officially become an adult. The glimmer of being able to stay up late, to eat whatever I wanted whenever I wanted, was so attractive to me. I could make my own rules and do whatever I wanted to in accordance with my own happiness. There was a promise of freedom and nothing but fun. Naturally, I thought adulthood would be like any playground game or exactly how it played out in any family movie. I would be neat and tidy; and at the end of it a cheesy song would play and we would all live happily ever after.

And then, like so many who are reading this book, I grew up, and thought to myself...really? *REALLY*?! This is it?! It's NOTHING like the movies! Truly, I quickly started wishing on days I could go back to being a kid.

Now, don't get me wrong, growing up and "adulting" does have its perks—technically, we can stay up late...barring any other responsibilities, of course. Technically, we can eat whatever we want...bearing in mind any health concerns, and maintaining a particular lifestyle aiming towards longevity. And, I suppose you could make up your own rules—so long as you are living within the law. Sure, there is freedom...to an extent, and if you're lucky there is a glimpse of fun. But let's be honest with each other—THIS STUFF IS HARD. And often, as adults, we do NOT have all of the answers!

No one plans for the hiccups of life; and no one warns you of heartache, disappointment, health concerns, roadblocks—that's never the narrative that is portrayed, and therefore, it is EFFING SCARY when life hits you with a couple of sour lemons. Who do you lean on, where do you go, and who can you trust? Your mind often runs a mile a minute, and sometimes it feels like a neverending hamster wheel.

There's no textbook or guide, no "how-to" on successfully adulting, or even how to navigate life as we experience it. All we really have is each other. And, actually, that's quite a bit - potentially everything we could need and want. **We have each other and our stories to lean on and learn from.** In a sense, this *is* the guide; the conversations we have, the connections we make, and, in continuing to show up boldly as our unique selves, like the true BOSSES we are.

And, while we truly cannot prepare for every second of every day—as part of life's magic is in the unknown—*Handling Hard Stuff (Like a BOSS)* follows the turbulent, yet triumphant journey of these everyday humans as they experience life as we do—putting one foot in front of the other, just trying to move forward in the best way they know how.

Sure, life can be hard—moments turning into memories, memories turning into pivotal points in our lifeline—but life isn't impossible (even though some days it may feel like it). While not every story ends with living happily ever after, or even comes to an end as a whole, the lessons and experiences we learn along the way are what makes the journey worthy.

The acceptance of the process—and the allowance of letting one feel each emotion through the rollercoaster of it all—is what makes you a BOSS. It isn't in finding a solution or tying up every bit in a neat little bow; it's the journey. The experience. It's getting dirty and experimental with life, and trusting yourself enough to wake up each morning, take a deep breath, and move forward, acknowledging that everything will turn out as it should.

Handling hard stuff (like a BOSS) is trust. It is self reflection. It is self-defining what being a BOSS is, taking pride in who you are and the experiences you have journeyed through. In our own way, we are each a BOSS; intrinsically the BOSS of ourselves and the way this crazy journey of life ends up.

My name is Sharana Ali, and over the course of several years I have grown a platform and a brand that centers around showing up for yourself and your life *unapologetically*. I began tapping into the power of authenticity, vulnerability and connection in 2018, sharing openly on my social platforms about what I was experiencing in my life, and hosting community events for humans desiring more depth from their relationships to themselves and others. My brand started becoming the go-to space for building upon these human desires, through the three pillars I established as important to accessing out potential: brunch, opportunities, and a support system. BOSS. (Boss in "the six", to be exact.) Through our combined love of great food, connection and community, BOSS events became safe spaces to turn taboo topics into table conversation. And then, an idea formed. I'd participated in a handful of collaborative writing projects and had become a published author in 2019, so I wondered... was there room for the women in my community to share their stories and life lessons?

As it turns out, yes, there was. *Handling Hard Stuff (Like a Boss)* is the culmination of this very thought. These women have practiced strength, courage, and bravery as they've taken their varying life lessons and experiences and turned them into beautiful, vulnerable, and authentic stories that have the power to heal. There is always space to be vulnerable, real, and authentic—and there is always a place to grow through what you go through... *like a boss.*

Happy reading,

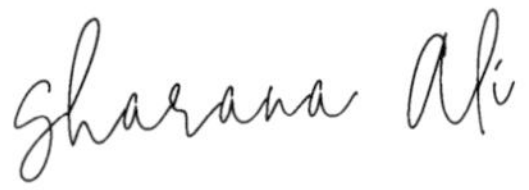

Lead Author, *Handling Hard Stuff (Like a Boss)*
Founder, B.O.S.S Network, @bossthesixedition

Chapter 1
ALI MARTIN

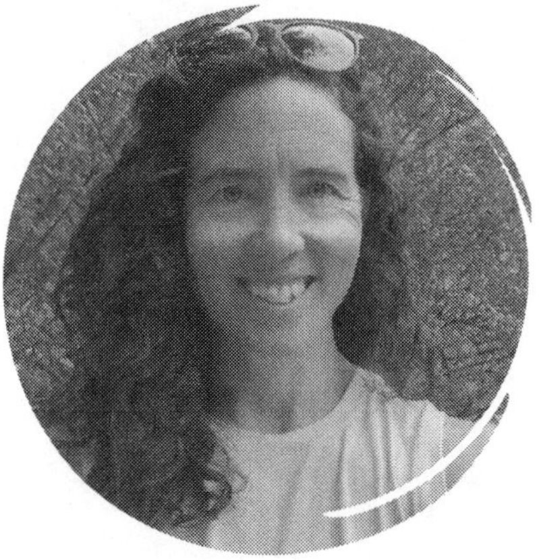

@ali_martin_

I've started writing this chapter about 27 times. Each time I start with confidence and direction, feeling good about the words that are flowing and my thoughts coming together in a way that might, just maybe, make sense to the reader. I mean, how the hell does one pull together words that could ever convey such matters of the heart? Especially when the story is about how a single decision changed the trajectory of my life, my kids' lives, and ended a relationship that, on paper, was gold. This chapter describes my "hardest thing," the process I took in coming to the decision that my marriage was no longer the relationship that I was meant for. I now see it as the catalyst for a lifetime of learning and re-learning, and something that, at times, feels equally difficult; ***the courage to listen to my heart and trust my decisions.***

Ever since I was a teenager I have carried this feeling around with me. I can remember feeling as though I was in the wrong place, that I was often misunderstood and could never quite accurately convey how I was feeling. As I say this, I am certain that this is part of growing up and that we all experience this "in-between" place of who we think we are and who we are meant to be. I had a deep understanding that my life was going to ask some very big things of me—experiences that would test my commitment to myself, the learning and leaning into who I am, and where my heart landed—over and over again. I've held on to that current of awareness, sometimes with excitement and other times with anxiety and hesitation over not wanting to make big things happen. It was easier to sit on the sidelines and just watch life go by instead of participating. I can vividly remember various levels of ignoring and avoidance, whether intentional or unconscious.

Eventually, the feeling got loud enough that it could no longer be pushed aside or accepted that "things were ok" the way they were. The most confusing part to me was that my life often looked and sounded like what I thought I wanted and "should" have been enough... but I couldn't deny that the time had come to pay attention and feel my way through the hardest things.

Fast forward 20 years, and I've had a few people ask me when I knew. Sometimes I feel an answer surface quickly, and other times I find myself trying to attach words to a feeling. How does one articulate the knowledge that ending a 16-year marriage to a great guy and an amazing Dad to our 2 kids was what I needed to do? The "right" thing to do? It was—and sometimes still is—the hardest thing that I've had to navigate up to this point.

I was 19 when we met. He was seven years older than me and felt like protection from day one. I was navigating my healing and recovery from personally challenging times, learning and re-learning about who I was within this new identity—and he felt like a knight in shining armour. Having him in my life gave me permission to lay down the swords that I held against myself and he would happily fight the demons for me. He was good at it, and I will be grateful until my last day that he was there to hold my heart as I started to mend the parts of myself that needed him. As I look back now, that dynamic served the purpose of belonging, connection, and being loved, but also robbed me of growing up in many ways. We fell in love and our story designed itself into a life that felt right for the people we were at the time. The chapters lined up in perfect order; we had great jobs, got married, bought a house, and welcomed two girls into our lives, 2 years and 10 months apart. Our rhythm of life was in sync and the months turned into years of "this is the rest of our life." At first that saying was a comfort, and then, eventually, I felt like I couldn't breathe, and it broke my heart.

The feeling dissipated for a while, sometimes years at a time. Life was rolling along in what felt like all the right ways and we settled into the roles that fit accordingly. As the days of making dinners, birthday parties, parent-teacher interviews, family trips, making sure the kids were taken care of, and trying to tend to our own needs wore on, I would occasionally hear this voice asking me, "Are you sure? Is this it? Is this how you are choosing to feel for the rest of your life?" I wouldn't let it stick around for long because it hurt to hear; it was terrifying to think that I would ever let myself believe that all that I had wasn't enough or where I was supposed to be. I was painfully aware of the confusion of why this didn't feel right. Why wasn't this enough? Why can't I just be grateful and happy and make my heart decide that landing here was what was supposed to happen?

Since then I have come to learn and love the fact that I WAS exactly where I was supposed to be in order to be where I am now. I got very frustrated at the fact that I couldn't come up with exactly what I was feeling or exactly what was wrong. I felt off; like a part of me was missing and I was being called from another place. I was aimless and felt empty at times, yet there I was, surrounded by the best of the best. There was huge hesitation to stare my life in the eyes and no longer feel that it was supposed to be mine. I started to live in a state of wanting to want it so badly, and it was exhausting.

I know that we have all tried to convince ourselves of something that we, deep down, know not to be true. It is depleting, stressful, and demands a lot from someone. This showed up for me in different ways. I was constantly on the verge of tears and my heart and head swirled in confusion. I would start a million different projects, hoping that they would provide a sense of completion and identity. I spent countless hours watching my life as an outsider and convincing myself that I was happy. At that point, letting it surface hurt too much and I couldn't see anything outside of my reality. My head would tell my heart that this reality was awesome and to look around at what I had, to not hurt the one I loved and knew loved me back, and that we were loving each other in the best way we could at the time.

I read book after book about love and the research on relationships, hoping to get an understanding of what I was feeling and ultimately get some answers. I played out hypothetical conversations with friends about the idea of being restless in a marriage and the eye rolling annoyances of their partner. None of what I was finding resonated with me. I was looking for external explanations for an internal issue.

Our relationship had always felt easy. We never fought—like, ever. While this kept the peace and made things smooth as the days passed by, it eventually felt as though there was a lack of opportunity to grow and evolve; not only for me as an individual, but as a contributing partner in a union. I was spinning my wheels and not getting anywhere, and it felt like there were many things missing—for myself and for him.

It felt comfortable because it was familiar, but the energy was stagnant and suffocating at the same time. Our friendship was strong and we had the ability to make the time pass in a way that appeared fulfilling. We always supported each other's decisions and I felt that there wasn't anything I could do wrong or be disagreed with in any way. He and I have talked in great detail about this since, and we have both learned and acknowledged that attachment styles influenced how we navigated our relationship from the beginning. It became my red flag and I even wrestled with that awareness! WTH… I wanted to fight!? I wanted turmoil and disagreements and rocky times?? I now understand that I wasn't having needs met that allowed me to feel as though I had something to grow up against—to have my mindset challenged and my heart opened to different angles of loving and being loved.

So much of what made me deny, distract, and turn inside out about all of this was the impact of my decision on our girls. Waves of feeling incredibly selfish to let myself think that I could, maybe, feel differently about my life at the cost of turning theirs upside down. To change their understanding of forever so that my version could feel more aligned and authentic. Looking back, I wonder how many hours I logged walking with that exact story in my mind. One foot in front of the other, trying to keep myself grounded as the tears were flowing and my heart dropped at the thought of having to put into words what I was feeling. I'd flip back and forth from trusting myself and my understanding of what was to come and blocking it all off, accepting that I could live and love this life as it was.

Amidst the emotional ping pong, a soft yet very powerful sense of knowing would reassure me with one sentence: *You can trust it; you will be okay and you will come to know how to endure the hard feelings.* This quiet understanding would somehow comfort me during the nights that I cried myself to sleep, the times a song would come on and I'd cry my eyes out on the side of the road, and the endless pages of notes I'd write as I tried to make sense of the shit that I was wading through. It allowed me to rest and trust and to not always feel as though I had to cognitively know the answer.

I had to trust myself in knowing that our girls would still be loved by the same parents and that we would do all that we could to navigate and build a new dynamic of parenting. I knew this of him and trusted myself in knowing that we would live that into existence. I had to trust that our kids were individuals—brave and capable girls who would integrate this experience, full of emotion, into that path that was theirs and only theirs. I would support, love, and hold them through it, but I couldn't make it anything other than what it was going to be for them.

I'll never forget the days leading up to when we were to share our decision with them. We spent many hours in conversation over how we hoped it would go and the various ways we were hoping to support their reactions. We went to therapy together and individually to best support ourselves and to create a language that we felt best fit our intentions and decision. We wanted to be as emotionally equipped as we could be for however it was going to unfold.

> ***"What we are teaches a child more than what we say, so we must be what we want our children to become."***
>
> *-Joseph Chilton Pearce*

Part of the inner knowing that haunted me was realizing that in order to honor myself, I had to confront some very hard decisions. To be able to say that I was showing up for myself and walking in the world as the person I needed to be, the girls were going to witness and be a part of my hardest decisions.

I wrestled with the guilt of this for a very long time before and after the fact. The action of my needs being met meant changing the course of the life they knew and felt safe in. This messaging took time to reframe and gain understanding around the bigger picture I was holding. I worked at the idea (with many hours spent with my therapist) and came to realize that it was knowledge I already had; my decision making wasn't going to ruin them. It was going to be an example of two respectful and compassionate adults making a very hard decision that honored and supported a life that looked different than the one they once shared. That didn't take away the love we had for the girls, the level of respect that he and I had for each other, or the commitment we had to parenting these two amazing kids as they grew into self-aware humans who could recognize how to do hard things.

I had to look at it all as though it was providing them with opportunity, rather than taking it away—opportunities that others told me I should have been shielding them from and to "suck it up and just stay together for the kids." I couldn't wrap my head around that being a better example for my kids than the one that was going to be hard but rooted in self-love and awareness. It became my mantra. There were many moments when I worried that I was being naive and that there was no way that "love was enough" regardless of what it looked like. Was I trying to fool myself that we could all come out of this as more aware and secure versions of ourselves?

I spent what felt like years trying to understand what was driving the dissolution of my marriage. Why couldn't I love what was in front of me? How could I be so selfish as to not embrace and appreciate what I have with this man? I wasn't happy and that was hard to admit. There was a deep feeling around my relationship not being fulfilled, and that stopped me from showing up the way I wanted to and should have been. I knew that I wasn't loving him the way he needed, wanted, and deserved to be loved. Yet, I couldn't find the path back to how it once felt between the two of us. To admit that I had outgrown the relationship and that my needs could no longer be met by him broke my heart. These were all things I fought with, feeling endless guilt around there being "nothing wrong" but my heart also knowing that it wasn't right. I knew that having things stay the way they were would break my heart in a different way, along with his. We had grown to the edge of us and I couldn't deny it.

I remember trying to think of specific events as to why this was the way I felt. Was there something that happened to me as a kid that I had forgotten and that made me not know how to accept love when it was staring me in the face? Had I missed out on learning about relationships because I only had one boyfriend before meeting him at 19? Maybe it was just the way relationships work and they all, eventually, get to a point where people just drift by each other because "it isn't that bad." I wasn't sharing my feelings and situation with very many people, mainly due to being exhausted from thinking about it AND out of fear of what people would think.

As I chose to share with a few very close friends, one supportive conversation stood out the most to me. My friend was empathetic and asked me, "How long can you be okay with just *okay*?" That question was posed for the both of us, and it was a pivotal point in my understanding of my heart's process. "Just okay" wasn't a concept that affected just me. It had become status quo for how I lived my days, how he did, and how our kids witnessed a marriage relationship. Sure, they saw their parents getting along and passing the days, but I knew that I wanted to set the example of their parents being the best versions of themselves... whatever that looked like. I hoped that, down the road, that would look like both of us honoring ourselves and having the courage to do hard things—for us to each be a part of a union that exemplified a bond that supported growth, love, and the ability to recognize (and undoubtedly fulfill) each other's needs.

Life as we knew it at that point was feeling unfulfilled, and we were coasting as "just okay." I was far from showing up in the ways that I wanted to be for him, and would resist when he tried to show up for me, after years of trying to be someone I couldn't access for us. Life is rich and vast and meant to be lived vibrantly from the heart, in between the mundane everyday stuff. I needed that for both of us—all of us.

Time passed, and the event of sharing with him where I was at with our life together happened late one Wednesday night. I had gone out for lunch with one of my closest friends and been in awe (not the cool kind) of the fact that I had once been at such a loss of knowing how to get to this place. She played a very big role in supporting me in ways that were non-judgmental, allowing me time, space, and a quiet place to be when I needed to be. Her trust in me helped me trust myself when I couldn't see past the fear. From the endless tears over having no clue how I was going to be brave enough to say anything out loud, to having the conversation with him, navigating that space of when one is leaning in and the other is leaning in a different direction, and spending a year still living together after having made the decision, we were preparing ourselves and intentionally working on what the change in dynamic between us was going to look and feel like.

The only way I could explain my arrival to that point in time was that I pushed myself to trust and feel my way forward—to trust that I'd know what to do. I would meet a feeling and invite it in, despite the pain and confusion that it brought. I would take deep breaths followed by processing it all in whatever way felt necessary at the time. Sometimes that meant sitting in silence or listening to my saddest playlist. Sometimes it looked like running through a forest, absorbing the strength of the trees through osmosis, or blasting the music and dancing in the kitchen after dinner. Sometimes it looked like sitting on the porch with a friend who knew the silence didn't need to be filled. And there I was... trusting my heart and scared shitless while doing so. I still am.

The space between the love that's shifted and the love that we are moving towards is where we meet ourselves. It takes us on one hell of a ride and the courage to hold on can be exhausting, but the sense of self and freedom is worth it.

Over the last five years I have met and re-met myself many times. I'd get lost in the worry that I had changed as a person—beyond who I even recognized—confused and tearful over the most recent heartbreak and terrified of not knowing how this story ends and who I wanted to be. I'd reach out to those closest to me and have reflective sounding board conversations and be gently (or sometimes, not so gently—gotta love those BLUNT besties) reminded that the core of who I am will never change. My virtues of respect, truth, compassion, self-honor, and discernment were still steering my ship, and to not know how it ends is called *having faith*. (I still question the comparison of faith and being naive, at times.)

Seeing the world through rose-colored glasses has tripped me up a few times, and it will again! But that part of me is always followed up by that same deep understanding that I am right where I need to be. I believe that my life is made up of a series of decisions that I can trust, and that when made from a heart-led, intentional place—can't be wrong.

This doesn't protect me from pain or heartache. It doesn't mean that my days are going to be blue skies and struggle-free from here on out; I fully understand that. But it does keep reminding me that I can trust my heart and know that I can handle the hard things, despite the fear and uncertainty. I am continuing to feel my way forward into new things, and my heart exhales with the knowledge that it has met a place that it can call my greatest adventure and home, all in the same breath.

We have watched and supported our girls through the last five years, ensuring lots of time and space for them to steer their own ships through their version of this experience. There have been moments of feeling confident and like award-winning calibre parents, and others where we have fumbled and dropped the ball, worrying that we've ruined them forever. Knowing that there are undoubtedly still hard times to come, we are grateful that the decision we made five years ago has become an example of trust, faith, and showing the importance of respect and unarmored conversation. He and I hold a true desire for each other to be happy and to be open and committed to new relationships and versions of ourselves.

I don't mean to gloss over the hardest times; please know that there have been MANY tearful and "WTF have I done?" moments. I have felt broken and cried myself to sleep on the floor of my kids' bedrooms after their Dad has come to pick them up. I have screamed into pillows, wandered around my neighborhood at 2:00 a.m., and stared at myself in the mirror searching for the finality of an answer. There have been dark times where I wished I didn't feel things as deeply as I did and could ignore the work involved in living a life true to myself. And through it all, I always come back to being thankful that I stay in commitment to myself.

I hold a great deal of gratitude that he was the other half of this. Without his open heart/open mind approach and his willingness to respect and try his best to understand me, I know this story would be very different. I am who I am, in a lot of ways, because of him.

I don't know where it comes from—my soul/heart/intuition/gut—but that feeling still arrives after the tears; it softens the uncertainty, lights up the darkness, and helps me find my feet. I am slowly comforted by that quiet understanding... I'm capable and committed to feeling my way forward and leaning into my most authentic life. I'm grateful for the experiences that have brought me to today and believe that we all have the capacity to trust ourselves; sometimes we just need to be shown the way back to knowing how.

Chapter 2
ASHLEIGH STEPHENS

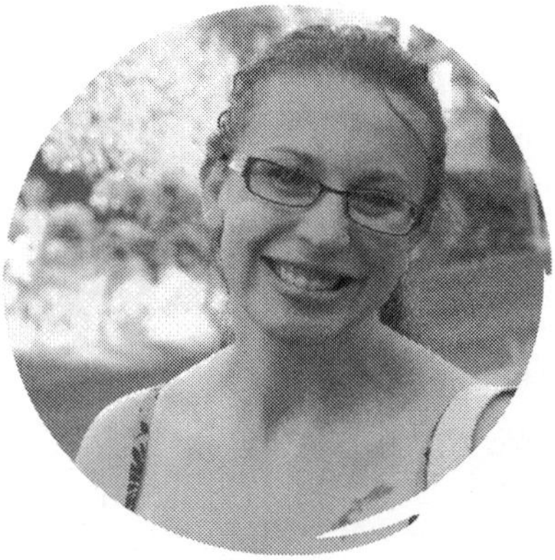

@ashleighstephens84

I sit here, propped up in my bed this evening. I won't lie; I've been lounging here since around 4:00 p.m. After coffee this morning, I jumped up, threw on yesterday's sweats, and mowed the lawn. I wanted a nice, clean-cut lawn before diving into planting all of the new perennials that I bought yesterday. I definitely overdid it a bit on my budget, but it's my first official spring in the new house. (I don't get the impression that the lady who lived here before me did much outdoors.) After a COVID winter and months spent launching my business, my physical fitness is lacking, to say the least, and I'm officially pooped.

Tomorrow is the Scorpio Full Super Moon, and it has me in a bit of a funk. Plenty of doubts, fears, and obsessive thoughts are coming into my awareness, but I've learned what to expect from any sort of Pluto-influenced transits. Perhaps you are wondering why this is a thing that I think about at all. Well, I'll tell you about it.

I took a deep dive into Astrology a few years back. And I guess when I say that, I should mention that it, as well as tarot, and all things woo-woo in nature, were right up my alley as a kid. At the age of 10, I began seeing things others did not perceive, and my adventure seemed to begin within the spiritual realm. It wasn't until a few years ago, however, that I began to revisit it once again. For a period of about 12 years, I let it all go... well, mostly. I had a real life to live, after all, and I was taking off on a trail to my own success. And that trail was that of marriage, family, and a career (and then, eventually, the destruction of most of it).

It hasn't been until the last few years that I have been able to look back and see how, as I diverted from being unequivocally me, I was setting myself up for quite the karmic lesson. It's one that, now, I rest truly grateful to have received. Be that as it may, the process was less than pleasant. In fact, it was downright heart-shattering.

When things began to disintegrate in my marriage, he became a person I no longer knew. People do that, you know? It happens. One day you're soul mates, and the next day they're telling everyone what a nasty person you are. They paint the picture the way they see fit. It doesn't matter if where they are coming from is completely accurate, or even truthful. Either way, they are going to survive this, come hell or high water, and whatever way gets them there is the road they are willing to blaze.

He not only called and spoke with his family about what happened between us, but he made his way down the call list and began calling mine. And for a brief moment, the part of me that wanted others to know that I'm not 100% at fault urged me to step in and defend myself. But by this time, I'd already spent hours upon hours with my ego, doing my best not to feed its narrative and dirty cries for hate-fire. So, instead, I sat in meditation. When I was angry and bursting at the seams to send all that pain in his direction, I said " ho'oponopono" instead.

I didn't hate him—far from it—and many nights, I went to bed after the girls went to sleep and lay there seething, letting the pain of it all rip me to shreds. Sometimes it was because I needed to feel sorry for myself—because as far as I could gather, no one else did. But more often than not, it was because I knew that the pain needed to have its way with me. If I let it tear me apart right now, it wouldn't try to come back later and do the same thing.

But I'm getting way ahead of myself. When I sat down to write this, I thought, hey, this will be cathartic and I'll get the chance to tell my story. Not because I need other people to know what horrible pain I've experienced as a result of this divorce process... no. Not because of that. But because I need to speak my personal truth, and I need just one person out there to know that while I was fighting the good fight, I was doing it for us both. I consciously decided that at some point, following the hell that I was about to embark my way through, I would someday have the words, the wisdom, and the lessons to share—making it so that I'm not doing this alone. I am doing it with you.

At that time, I wrote maybe three paragraphs and set it aside. How am I going to compartmentalize this experience into a single chapter? How am I going to write this the "right" way, and not in an ugly way that no one deserves... but somehow also honors my truth?

Well, today is four days until the anniversary of my divorce being finalized. It seems that after a year of being on my own, a single mom, and a whole mess of other events, including a global pandemic, now feels like the right time to get it out.

So, yeah... in a way, we did this process together. You and I. To the person reading this—I hope this finds you as well as can be expected. You aren't alone. You are understood; and my heart goes out to you and this uniquely terrible yet beautiful experience can be something we always share, even if we never speak.

When I first met Sean, our relationship was already considered taboo. It was right around the time that online dating was still considered a faux pas. I think that's part of what made it so exciting; we were defying the odds from the get-go. I knew I was crazy about him within days of our constant back and forth chatting, and at the point that we graduated to webcam, his smile and his intense interest in getting to know me was both a relief and very exciting. I'd spent my whole life feeling like an oddball. Most people I know would probably think that sounds funny to them, because I was definitely social, definitely outgoing, and definitely confident. But there had always been something lacking—some untouchable, unidentifiable thing—and I always felt like I was weird. I saw things differently. The things that I found interesting were not interesting to anyone else I knew at the time.

Sean and I officially met in person on Labor Day weekend in 2006. I instantly felt at home. All the nervousness I expected to feel wasn't there; it was all just excitement to finally see one another. To finally touch. To laugh together and it not be interrupted by a bad wifi connection. There was something about him that just fit right to me. I loved that he wasn't nervous either. I loved that he was also excited. I loved that he was already so steady, so affectionate, so warm. It was as if our handful of weeks talking online or over the phone had already played the part of the weird beginning stages of a relationship... only it never felt weird then, either. He felt safe. Rock solid. He was terribly intelligent, loved to laugh, loved to hold my hand, and was completely comfortable being silly with me. It was like magic—the kind you forgot you knew, but when it arrived, it was like riding a bike.

By the end of the long weekend, I knew we needed to be together. We were a match. I'd finally found my person, someone that fit with me and I with them. The small act of separating and going back to our lives after such a short time together was a heartbreaking experience. I know that sounds odd to anyone else; we'd only just met. We'd only been talking for about two months. And normally, it wouldn't have made sense. But with Sean, it just did, and something about that felt divine. Destined. Something so perfectly matched that only the gods could have pulled it off. He was handsome. He was sweet. He was the most unconditional person I'd yet to meet.

For a period of about three months, we took turns traveling the roughly 500 miles to see one another—driving, flying, meeting in the middle. Home didn't really feel like home after that. Home was with Sean. So before Christmas rolled around, I found a job near him, put in my notice, and packed a truck full of my things. He came down to help me drive the truck back to Iowa, to our first apartment together.

We were married four years and a week after meeting. Had it not been for everyone's Labor Day weekend plans, that would have likely been when we chose our date. Instead, we went with the following weekend. By then, we'd already lived in two rentals and had bought our first fixer-upper. While all that wasn't the top of my list, we'd already accomplished a lot together. Anything we did together didn't stand a chance. We'd already discovered that before marriage: if we were on the same team, nothing could stand in our way. And boy did we have plans.

With both of us coming from divorced parents, we knew that marriage was a big, important step that needed to be carefully approached. We knew we wanted to have kids. By the time we'd chosen a date to marry, I'm not sure what we were more excited about—getting married or starting our family, our way.

This is not to say that the entire four years leading up to marriage was easy. It wasn't. For a lot of it, we struggled to make ends meet. If it wasn't a cheap enough spot to live, the heating bills would kill us. When I moved up, he was in school and I took a major pay cut. We did a lot of things to stretch the budget, but we were always in it together. Our ideas of fun were sometimes different than what others were doing. We did a lot of things that didn't cost money. We did a lot of exploring. We made a lot of memories instead. When marriage was approaching, we were finally making headway, gaining momentum in our careers, and climbing our way out of the poverty of college kids.

While I suspect that everyone's wedding day is a whirlwind, ours was as well. But the thing I recall most was that we had sealed the deal. We were now not just soulmates; we were family. I had every hope that we would survive anything life threw our way, no matter how crazy. So while the photos were being taken, I was his wife. When the toasts were happening, I was his wife. When the dancing started and the champagne was poured, I was his wife. We were bound together, and in so many ways, that sounds like a prison sentence. That's not how I felt. When I say bound, it was a chosen sentence—one that meant to us and to others that we were together and we could handle anything.

We were wrong.

Within a month's time, I became pregnant. Within five month's time, I was laboring and giving birth to our dead son. I woke up on February 13th to one huge contraction, and it broke my water. By Valentine's Day, he was gone and I felt completely dead inside, wondering why I couldn't have just died with him. The mourning began before he even arrived. We went first to the ER, then a hospital bed. Then we had a meeting with the doctor and got the news that this was all over. We made a quick trip home to gather some things for a hospital stay. We sat on that front porch step, knowing that by the time we returned home again, my womb would be empty and so would our arms. We made a move to a different hospital. The nurses spent hours just attempting to get me into labor and I felt like all I could do was lay there, knowing that his heart still continued to beat, knowing that I was getting my last few hours with him. It seemed I was in the hospital bed, watching TV, lost in a daze of absolute despair, while everyone else around me was aflutter and in constant movement. Sean welcomed our parents, one at a time. At one point I recall him being concerned that I might die there, along with the baby, because the longer my water was broken without labor, the higher the risk for infection grew. They pumped me full of antibiotics and pitocin, but it continued to be a slow process.

As I think back on it, I think that was somehow my doing. And the baby's. There was no more amniotic fluid, and per the ultrasound, he lay curled into the fetal position, heart still going strong. It's as if somehow we both knew our time together was ending, so his heart kept going and my labor refused to progress—like we both chose that for a night, we'd stop time and spend it together. I'm certain my memories of that experience are flawed. I was in shock and the trauma was cutting me in half. But what I do know is that I decided to choose a Disney movie on the hospital TV and I watched it with him, my hand on my stomach...because no one was going to take that small thing away. When the movie did end, the nurses came in to talk to me about what the process would be like—that he may be born alive, as his heart just kept beating, to everyone's surprise except mine. When they left the room, I began to pray. I knew if he was born alive, that would be what killed me. The thought of him suffocating to death was more than I could handle. So I prayed like my life depended on it. I didn't just pray, I threatened God or what I knew of him/it. I prayed to my dead grandfather, begging him to come escort him home. I prayed to the baby, asking him to go ahead and let go. If he left now, he could pass away safe in my womb and not be subjected to the madness that seemed to exist just outside of my body.

Then the labor progressed all at once. He was born, and had thankfully passed away before arriving. Regardless of my grief, I exhaled knowing that. They wrapped him up and handed him to me. He was tiny. He was frail and tiny. It felt like a shock to my entire being—the same weight in my hands was the exact weight that had just been in my womb. And finally, everyone left us for the night. I placed him in a crib next to my bed. Sean slept in the horrible hospital chair turned fold-out cot. I wouldn't allow them to take him away. At some point, he was baptized. Just before they had me leave the hospital, they took him away to the nursery... promising me they would handle him with care and see him cremated. It took me an hour just to go inside our home. Crossing the threshold without him felt too final. Within days my lactation began and I was officially a broken mother without a baby. It felt like a curse to be a woman, fully prepared to nurse a new baby, and he was nowhere to be found. Only a mother knows what I mean when I say this: when a baby arrives, your body returns to its animal nature; you're just the observer of the process. I felt like a caged lion. Like a mama elephant who'd just lost her baby to poachers. I was a mother. A babyless mother.

The weeks that followed were pretty bittersweet and horrific. I cried more than I think I ever have in my life, before then and still until now. Sean was hurt and we took solace in one another. For a time, his heart was open and he was gentler than he'd ever been. It didn't feel like long before he was angry with my continued sorrow. He said and did things that changed us forever. It changed how I viewed him, and my respect for him was broken. He didn't want to mourn; he'd tired of the process, and when I continued to feel like hell, he grew angry with me because of it. I grew angrier with him for behaving heartlessly, for referring to our lost child as "not a real person." I can look back at it now in a different light: I was a mama bear, somehow feeling the need to defend a lost baby from his own father, and he was just lost. Both of our dreams had been shattered in short order. The honeymoon phase of our marriage was not only over, but it had been set on fire. After a couple of months, the best my doctor could do was tell us to try again, and hand me a script for Xanax. I took one half of a pill from the entire bottle; drugs to numb me out wasn't what I was after. I just wanted something I couldn't have—to not have lost a child and to not have lost my respect for Sean.

Our second child arrived a year later. That process, while successful, was also very trying. We avoided announcing the pregnancy until after the 17 week mark; that felt like a mark in time that needed to be accomplished first. By 26 weeks, I was put on hospitalized bed rest because low back pain turned out to be labor. I was fully effaced and dilated 2 centimeters. We were back in complete terror and I wasn't sure we were going to catch a break. To the shock of all the nurses and doctors, the contractions did finally stop, days into the horrendous drugs they were trying on me. I spent Christmas, New Years, and several more weeks in the hospital, just praying that my water didn't break.

I was caged up in a hospital room, facing my worst fears with each passing moment, while Sean drove back and forth the 40 miles from home to see me most days. We argued a lot. I was mad at him and he at me; we were each other's easiest targets.

Fast forward another four years, and our second daughter was born healthy, and this time with medical encouragement, as it seemed she would have remained happily in my womb forevermore. It was a shocking change of events after the first two, but I wasn't complaining! Thus far, Sean and I had been through quite the rollercoaster ride within our marriage, and now our expanded family. We had high highs and the lows were some of the lowest. Overall, however, we were all healthy, our budget was a far-cry from fresh out of college, and our careers had steadily been on the rise for some time. We, technically speaking, had it all—a big house, nice cars, family, friends, health, and abundance. What we hadn't figured out was why that was still unsatisfactory. What we did figure out was that when all of life's obstacles finally gave us some room to breathe, our survivalist mentalities and our unstoppable teamwork transformed into opposing forces, looking for problems in one another.

Now, I'd say that for the most part, I've lived my life as a good person. In the grand scheme of things, I've spent very little time in the dark, throwing my ugliness at others. Conversely, most of my life I've taken charge, pulled the troops together like a mother hen, and worked my ass off to ensure that all responsibilities were covered. I've worked hard and spent the time I should have been playing caring for others, helping others, or standing up for others. When others would seemingly crumble in the face of adversity, I hardened up and fought the good fight. The only problem was that I often felt that I knew best, and when challenged, this hardened leader had a habit of turning her blunt and brutal determination towards those I had been fighting to protect.

At some point, I decided to really look at just how hardened I'd become. I had a gift of internal fire that was so strong, it was out of my control. I didn't like how overpowering it could become, but I was aware that it had a proclivity to injure others—and that wasn't who I wanted to be. I'd also, honestly, tired of hearing about my brutal nature from others, and well, if I could fix it, they wouldn't be left with much to complain about. And so began my journey into myself. I raise my hat to those who had the ability to break down those walls; there was nothing short of a miracle that would have gotten through to me at that point—all except my intense love for those that showed me a mirror—Sean being towards the top of that list.

And so the self-reflection began: meditation, exploring my triggers, and a lot of deep, dark work on insecurities. By the time that I had experienced a full-blown spiritual awakening, I was already well on my way to distancing myself from the people I knew best. And this wasn't because I didn't care for them. It was because we started to lack a common connection. As it turned out, my deep dive into my own monsters was too late for Sean, and he had zero desire to join me in that kind of healing. Sean wasn't the least bit interested in my methods, my spirituality, or even the person I was becoming. The more he projected at me, and the less he was interested in working on it, the less I wanted to play the part of his target. Rather than being ashamed of my "downsides," they became parts of me that I loved, not because they were perfect and not because they didn't need work—they did—but because they ultimately helped me to survive up until this point. Who was I or anyone else to reject a fragment of me that helped me get to where I am today?

We often hear the saying, "Hindsight is 20/20." I agree with this sentiment. We can always look back and see what took shape and how, and often we do so with a tinge of regret for having not seen it clearly the first go-round. After what felt like a lifetime of one traumatic event after another, I was pretty fed up and irritated with hindsight. I mean, there had to be a way to really dive into a situation and come out with something better than simply normal human vision abilities. That really got me thinking about said conundrum. I had a really hard time believing that we were just meant to walk through life stepping into minefields, tumbling along like uprooted weeds in a desert. That was not only a depressing outlook, it was also extremely disempowering. So I decided to make it my goal to look so deeply into my own insecurities, my own faults, and my own contributions to my own misfortunes that by the time I came up for air, my vision was closer to that of a hawk: 20/2. With hindsight that intensely strong, there was no way I would walk around waiting for life to happen to me. I was tired of being a tumbleweed. It was high time my power was exactly that: my own. So that's what I did.

I did it for me. And when the descent into my own darkness was so dank and ugly that I didn't think I could handle any more of it, I pushed through it for my daughters. And when I kept crawling on my hands and knees through the muck, and it got harder still, I did it for you. When my personal will would waver, I'd find a new rope, tie it around my waist, and throw it into the future. Admittedly, this often happened as a way to distract myself from the clear fact that, free will or not, I was down in the darkness and no one was coming to rescue me. They couldn't if they tried, because this was my journey. Had I actually allowed myself to wobble and give up, finding it too brutal and repulsive, I'd have just laid there in the mud and wasted away.

The experience was ugly, and still, today, remnants arise that require my tender, loving care. I was not only facing my personal demons, but I was doing so while grieving a person

I had been completely sure was "my person." On top of that soul-tearing experience, that same person was busy smearing me at every turn, to anyone who held a bored but intrigued ear. They were people who likely felt like they were being supportive, so I grieved them as well. That same "soulmate" was whole-heartedly rejecting me, and it was a "me" that finally felt like my real self, not some societally created version that felt more palatable. All I could really seem to focus on, however, was not actually dying, protecting my girls as best as I could, and, eventually, coping with physical symptoms that danced in and out of PTSD or ego death.

When you look at a marriage that doesn't "make it" to death do us part, you can look at the ways in which you contributed to its ending. You can look at the ways in which the other spouse failed to uphold their end of the bargain. And if I had to guess, that's the approach most would take. Some take the really easy route and walk on, into their future, convinced that the entire problem was the other person. Well, I'm not most people, and I've never been quite satisfied with the status quo. In fact, whether Sean was completely to blame for the entire thing, I was going to walk the path as if it were all me from the start. And not from the start of the marriage... no, no. I was going all the way back to the very beginning. I was going back to baby Ashleigh. Now, I know our ended relationship, filled with both happiness and terror, wasn't all me. That's not possible and only can be now as I sit here, single and free.

You see, there's a real, solid choice here. And in my lifetime, it's probably the most solid choice I've ever encountered. The kind that's absolutely a fail-safe option. There's no way to fail this one! The only way to mess this up is to choose option B or C. So now you're wondering, what's option B or C?! Well, option B is that you accept what you did mistakenly, and accept what they did mistakenly. Unfortunately, this option is open to interpretation and most people will walk away with only 20/20 hindsight here, continuing to tumble into minefields in the future (most of them with their injured hearts caged up behind steel doors for protection). Option C, an even poorer choice, is to blame it all on the other spouse. It sure feels good to the ego to do so, but I can almost guarantee you'll walk right back into the same scenario with a new person. Option C is for the victims of the world, the ones who haven't quite had enough time in the torture chambers of life. And please note, this is not a harsh judgment. My heart aches for those who choose as such, for I was, once upon a time, an Option B or C kind of gal.

Here's Option A: own it all. The entire shebang. Be completely and 100% responsible for what happened, no matter who did what, and own it. Now, as I write this, I can already read the bubbles over some of your heads: "Say what?! But it wasn't *all* my fault!" I can assure you, you are correct. However, when we place power in others, that's who has it. And that becomes a really slippery slope, because so long as you're not completely responsible, you'll remain floating on the whims of others, bobbing this way and that. If it's all about you and your responsibility, well... you'll have hawk-like hindsight and some phoenix-rising-level foresight as you finally step into the present moment. That doesn't mean that life will suddenly be all cherries and rainbows; I think we all know better than that. But what it can look like is this: You enter into relationships of all kinds, consciously—with an open heart and an open mind—knowing who you are and what you're worthy of and willing to tolerate. When you inevitably get punched in the gut, you rise again, just like the phoenix. Problems exist! Of course they do! But they don't need to be life-shattering experiences. Because now, you're a fully responsible and fully empowered, flawed, amazing human being.

In this way, every time you get upset, emotional, and devastated (and that will happen—a lot!) you can ask yourself these questions:

"Why did I do that?"

"Why did I enable that?"

"What part of me accepted that?"

"What do I know now?"

"What's the new story that I'm going to tell about that, if only to myself?"

"What advice would I give to my best friend in the same situation?"

"What advice would I give to my daughter in this situation?"

"How did I allow my personal power to step outside of myself in that situation?"

"What's the more empowered option?"

"If I were to love myself unconditionally in this very moment, what would I say to myself?"

And there's another superb bonus to Option A! When choosing this approach, you're spending time to reflect on your bad habits, self-sabotage tactics, and all that seemingly cringeworthy baggage. It's so hard to really have a look at that (in fact, it's downright ego-crushing). But, on the other hand, you've done the hard work, and anyone who isn't willing to do so, need not apply. Because suddenly, if you can do it, you emanate a requirement that others do the same. Not in a harsh, controlling, demanding kind of way, but in a loving, warm, and empowered kind of way. You just simply will not accept anything less than what you deserve (which, by the way, is absolutely everything your heart is capable of desiring).

After the eye-crossing dive into your own personal hell has left you both exhausted and blissed out at just how miraculous you actually are—warts and all—there's another wonderful reflection to try (this one much less heavy than the first, I promise). That is to look back and take full responsibility for all of the GOOD that happened as well. Sure, your spouse or significant other was there, sharing in the bliss. And sure, they also contributed. But I think you might find that some of your happiest, most beautiful moments were *you*... just shared with someone else.

And that is the real reward! Because not long after you've concluded that you were both your grief *and* your bliss—the entire time—you're suddenly and miraculously your own sovereign and powerful person. You no longer seek outside of yourself for happiness, because it's what you are. You no longer judge others, because you know what it is to be disempowered and in pain. Sharing experiences with others is suddenly the goal—not because you need to put your power out there to experience fulfillment, but because who wouldn't want to share an overflowing cup of wonderful? And then, suddenly, your grief for what once was dissipates. Any last remnants of anger or blame drift away on the breeze, and you find gratitude for the journey and where it's landed you today: loving yourself and the sight of a hawk, to boot. The naysayers and the shit-talkers become a mix of amusement and pity, because you know who *you* are—and that's actually all that matters.

I do want to say a few things before we wrap this up that I think you'll find are extremely important on your journey. One is to remember to love yourself, unconditionally, throughout the entire process. A lack of unconditional love of self is almost entirely why you're here to begin with, so love all of you and hold and nurture the parts of you that feel ugly and rejected. Secondly, allow yourself the space to make more mistakes or tumbles. It's okay. Just keep trying—for yourself and only you. If you were meant to be complete perfection, you probably wouldn't be here. Tip #3 is that while this is 100% responsibility of self, that doesn't mean that you're doing this alone, nor do you have to! Seek assistance from trusted sources, both professional and spiritual, or whatever best fits your situation. I wasn't kidding when I said that I did this for you. Anyone that takes such a personal and grief-stricken journey will know that it's not for the faint of heart, and it's not necessary to do it alone (if that can be avoided). And finally, thank you from the bottom of my expanded heart. I really couldn't have made it this far if I hadn't conjured you within my mind, knowing that this journey would serve even just one other person.

Now, go find that bad-ass within!

Chapter 3
CHANTAL CARRUTHERS

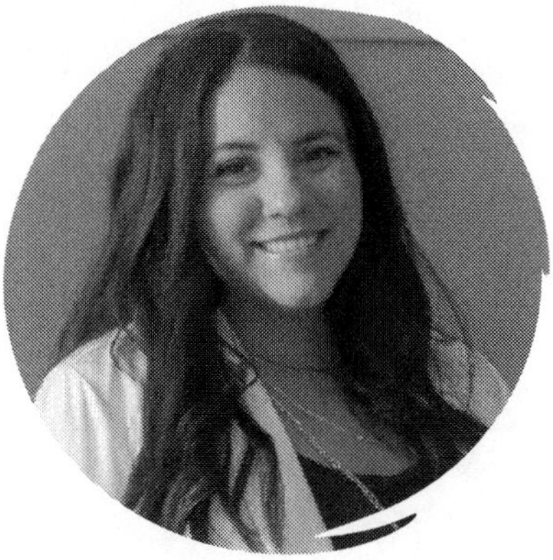

@Xchantillylacex
c_carr00@hotmail.com

Don't Underestimate Your Impact

When you hear something repeated over and over again, it can sometimes be hard to tune out. Our actions and our words define who we are. They tell our story, they shed light on our truth, and they express how we feel in the moment. Whether they are positive or negative, they can be powerful, inspirational, and influential, but can also be hurtful, deceitful, and full of lies. If you were to ask yourself, *are my words full of love and good intention or are they not?* What would your answer be? Maybe it's that they are a bit of both, but the downside is that they can be the start of a takeover for someone. That someone was me, and it was in the worst way. I never even imagined it was possible. I mean, how could somebody else's words dictate my life and force me to feel something that I didn't personally already feel? How could said words be so dominant over my very own thoughts, that I would allow a change in perspective of myself?

Our minds and our hearts evaluate people's words and, for some, they can ignore the hatred and move on because they know better. But when something happens repeatedly, it can lead us to thinking that there's truth behind it. That was also me. I would catch myself in moments realizing that I was repeating horrifying things to myself, and I was starting to believe it all. Despite those growing insecurities, there was so much more going on. We struggled immensely at times as a family. I experienced things that I wouldn't wish on anyone, but we made it through, as most of us do, when we experience bad things on our journeys through life. Most of our family struggles revolved around my mother and her health over the years. I watched her become a version of herself that she constantly said she didn't recognize. She would reminisce on the days when she wasn't so sick all of the time, when she wasn't overweight. She often felt insecure and, well, I couldn't help but allow those uncharted feelings to penetrate my own life, with the help of other people around me, of course. These people didn't seem to make anything easier at the time. But as a family, we experienced loss, and I got defeated, but I also found love and a new meaning to life. I am so grateful for that.

If more than one person around you says something about you, could there be truth to that? I always felt that it must take a "trained" mind to navigate those feelings in a healthy way, but sometimes, in the thick of it, something takes over and we go on believing this nonsense. Somehow we believe that somebody else knows better than our own self, and they go on dictating our worth by our successes—or in my case, my appearance—my weight, in particular.

It wasn't until I decided to really think back and dig deep, that I realized just how unprocessed these feelings were and how they still made an appearance from time to time. I grew up with a lot of self-doubt and heavy insecurities, just longing for acceptance and suffering from loneliness. I continued to fall deeper into this spiral of destruction even when I felt that I had already reached the bottom. I couldn't imagine things getting any worse. I often questioned myself: *Am I good enough? Do I deserve this life? How much longer will I need to endure this?* I constantly battled this uncomfortable feeling that there was nowhere I would be understood or accepted unless I lost weight. I would sit and cry alone, feeling trapped in this cycle all the time—more often than I ever let on to anyone.

The only way out for me was to fight it off and go on with my daily life, just acting like it never happened, or acting like I didn't care. I played tough and faked being okay most of the time. Some days I was, but others crippled me and had me feeling so out of control. Any insecurities I had would come flooding back. I'd get home from school and immediately break down. I'd scream terrible things to myself. I'd hate looking in the mirror and I'd have to start rebuilding myself again for the next day.

I was only in elementary school when it started, and some days were worse than others. At age 11, I was diagnosed with a condition called osteomyelitis (a bone infection) in my left femur. It was a lot to cope with at the time, but after a few terrifying weeks in the hospital, the conclusion was that it was treatable, and I was grateful for that. However, I was away from school for about a month as I continued to recover. When I returned to normal life, everything seemed to have changed. The bullying began surrounding my weight and I didn't even understand why there was such a sudden change in everyone's opinion on the matter. It even escalated to someone trying to set my hair on fire once. I was only in grade 7. I mean, am I the only one, to this day, asking myself *WHO THE HECK DOES THAT TO SOMEONE... EVER?* What did I do to make someone feel like they needed to do that to me?

I didn't feel like I should be ashamed of who I was. I felt like I had so much more to offer than what I looked like, but the hardest part for me was that I still had boyfriends, I still felt pretty despite being heavier, and I did feel good enough and deserving, so I was really confused as to why so many people insisted that I wasn't worthy of happiness. Some of these people were supposed to be my friends—or so I thought. I was so hurt, and when I look back, I still can't believe how hard people were on me... and especially how hard I was on myself. I was longing to be part of a group of people that would never understand me or appreciate me anyway. I couldn't stand for what they did. I didn't want those people as friends, and they were never going to offer me happiness in life. It was for the best that their actions pushed me further away from them, but it just grew from feeling sad and misunderstood to feeling tormented and angry.

I became really guarded and outspoken. I felt like I needed to defend myself constantly, and over time, I didn't pay any attention to how my words would possibly affect someone else. I was hurting other people the way I had been hurt. I didn't fully understand what positive relationships were. I was overshadowed with grief, and my actions were tarnished with resentment. I often implied that I didn't care what people were saying, that I had "thick skin," or that I was going to be my own version of myself despite their nastiness. I wasn't prepared to cope with all of that buildup. It went on for a good 4-5 years and I wasn't mature enough to properly store it away, if you know what I mean. During that time, when I felt at my lowest, fighting to break myself from this cycle, I felt like I didn't have anywhere to fall. You'd think that at such a young age I'd be able to go home and speak to my parents about it, but there was a whole new set of challenges there. Of course you hear the saying, "you never know what someone is going through, so be kind," but little did these bullies know, I had so much more going on behind closed doors. What they wanted to dish out to me was nothing in comparison.

I can remember being told that my mother was involved in a car accident when I was very young—two or three years old, if I can recall correctly. In and around the year 2000, she developed a very rare condition. It was never diagnosed, but she was suffering from severe neck pain and what started as a small coin-sized scab on the back of her head eventually turned into a large open wound covering the back portion of her scalp. She lost all of her hair in that area, it bled a lot, and it caused her pain. She endured countless doctor's visits and no one could identify what this was, what was causing it, or how to fix it. It was accompanied by migraines, neck and back pain, you name it—and so all of this started the beginning of trial and error prescription medications. Mostly everything she tried didn't work. She was a guinea pig. It turned into prescribing things that would simply make this way of living more tolerable, more comfortable, but it wasn't a solution or a way of healing. She eventually had to stop working due to the pain and side effects of the medications. It came down to her falling ill, bedridden for weeks at a time, and then she would just seem to get back up like nothing happened and resume her version of "normal." It was that way my whole life. I was so accustomed to seeing those wavering moments with her health. Sometimes she was even in and out of the hospital, but she always came back to us.

Through all of that, I remember my father working double time in order to continue to provide for our family, but we still struggled. We were a family of six, after all. I remember overhearing conversations about the possibility of us losing our home if they couldn't pay the bills on time, or when we would go short periods with no hot water and had to boil water on the stove to have our baths. It was that or the food on the table. Financial strain is a serious thing, and it can be so destructive. I know there were times when I didn't think their marriage could sustain any longer, but they fought through it to try and make a better life for us. I can honestly say, though, that it was hard for us to hear and even harder for us to watch. We watched them go from being so in love to feeling so disconnected over the years.

Considering my mom was home a lot, we built a very close connection. She was very involved—sometimes too much—but she was always very supportive. Regardless of her ongoing health concerns, she had a strong personality accompanied by an infectious smile. People adored her. She had an overwhelming love that flowed from within her and a constant need to give to others, even when she could barely afford things for herself.

Bearing in mind that I knew she was feeling distant in her marriage, I really saw a change in her when her first grandchild entered the world. It's almost as though my niece gave her a new way of feeling needed. She gave her a new purpose. My sisters and I were more grown up and more independent at that point, and she knew that this little person could depend on her. Spending time with her granddaughter reignited a joy in her life, and now that I am older and have children of my own, I can finally, truly appreciate that relationship—especially because, at age 19, on Boxing Day 2006, we lost her.

She had lost the battle with her health, and her once-radiant light had permanently faded. It was and still is the hardest thing

I have ever endured. I was moving into adulthood and making life-changing decisions, and I needed her. Why did this have to happen now, like this? I felt so lost, and I felt like her passing had happened so fast. She went into the hospital, and only a month and a half later, she was just gone—that was it. She was only 51 years old. She was going to miss out on every single one of my milestones moving forward... milestones that I know she would've been so proud to be a part of.

Unfortunately, as I started to encounter these moments, I constantly felt an emptiness that I knew would never be the same. It was only a short three years after she passed, that I started my relationship with my now-husband, and I know that she would approve of him! But she missed us buying our first home, she missed me picking my wedding dress and getting married, and the part that will always hurt the most is that she missed out on watching her grandchildren enter the world. I know they would've been her greatest joy. As tears roll down my face, I tell myself that time always heals—but with Mom, I truly miss her more and more as I continue living this life without her.

Every time I hear one of her favorite songs, or when I see something that reminds me of her, when Christmas rolls around, or especially when I'm tucking in my little ones with a blanket that she made, I miss her more. I could truly talk about her for hours. I can dive into how much of an influence she was for me, and what I learned from her. I find myself comparing who I have become, to her, frequently. I find my strength in her, and it's shaped me into the woman I am today.

Watching her fight off her insecurities as I grew up seemed like they became my own, but I—with time and the right mindset—learned how to let go of all of the hurt, pain, and shame that I had surrounding who I was and the body I was in. I was able to acknowledge that it wouldn't hold me back anymore. It was about time that I started accepting that I was deserving of living my best life in whatever body I had. I didn't have to feel guilty or scared of what others would say about me, because I had endured enough. I had wallowed enough. I had things to be grateful for, and it was time to acknowledge that. I couldn't let my lack of self-confidence control me anymore. Years of bullying, years of destructive talk, years of being overshadowed by confusing love examples had truly worn me down.

I could never be more grateful for the man I call my husband. He entered my life at just the right time. I was still mentally recovering from the damage, but he showed me what true love looked like. I was twenty-one. Any and all of the uncertainty I had slowly faded. I really do believe that "when you know someone's right for you, you know." There is no wavering.

We got married after 8 years together. We were blessed with two children and the rest is history. He was the one person who made me feel beautiful again. He was the one who made me feel worthy of love, and the one who showed me that all of those other opinions of people who didn't even take the time to know me—didn't matter. I was finally able to take my own life back. My self-confidence slowly crept back, too. I knew that my size shouldn't matter, but he proved that it didn't. I knew that I had more to offer people in my life than what I looked like. If someone wants to make fun of me because of my size, shame on them. I don't need to tolerate that, and it speaks volumes to what type of person they are. If that's you, I don't want you anyway. I truly hope for everyone that we choose the people who surround us, and they should be there because they bring a positive, honest, and genuine light in your life. The ones who don't aren't for you.

With all of that mindset recovering I was finally doing, insert pregnancy. It was a whole new experience for which I was ready, but not fully prepared. It brought on a whole new set of questions, a whole new perspective of my body and how it should look or would look, and a whole new set of expectations. It was a brand new thing that had the potential to make me question myself. But I had to acknowledge what it was doing. I suffered from HG (hyperemesis gravidarum) with my first pregnancy. Thankfully I was spared its terrible side effects for the last three months of my pregnancy, but it was quite a challenge. I had a relatively normal pregnancy otherwise. I was finally recovering from having this human evacuate my body, finally feeling more like myself—well, an extremely exhausted new version of myself that most moms can relate to—but insert pregnancy number two!

Our daughter was only three months old when we found out we were pregnant again. I felt like I went limp at the time and literally sobbed for days. I remember calling a friend of mine, before even talking to anyone else, and asking them how on earth I was supposed to do this. She reminded me that I was capable. I needed to hear it, in that moment, because I honestly just felt like my whole world had stopped. I started doubting the possibility that I could even overcome this. I couldn't imagine doing this all over again. This body that I had had so much shame around my entire life... was it going to sustain this?

I didn't feel ready in body or mind, but it was happening whether I was ready for it or not. If I wasn't going to have my mother there to convince me that everything was going to be okay, then my support system would be there, alongside my husband, of course. He always instilled peace in what was happening. He reminded me that he knew we were going to be just fine. I remember thinking about what my mom would've said to me at that moment. I can't say I know what her words would've been, but I definitely know that she would've helped me no matter what.

I asked myself, *how in the world am I going to raise these two babies without her help*? It once again hit me that I was going to have to live through something else in her absence... and this was something big. I mean, if you had any questions regarding your babies, who would you ask? How many people, as long as they are still blessed with the presence of their mother, would say, "my mom"? I believe that would likely be the most common response. She was supposed to share all of her insight and knowledge with me. She was the one who was supposed to know all of the home remedies for when my babies got sick. She would understand what these sleepless nights felt like, and would be there to take over for me when I felt too exhausted to keep going. But all of that was still gone. I mean, I had support from other people, but there is something most comforting about your own mother. There is no filter, no sugar coating, no pleasing—just truth and support. I know I would've appreciated that.

Despite discussing how hard I thought all of this was, I know that I am so lucky to have been able to have my own children, and I promise I will never take them for granted. I am so incredibly fortunate to have had no problems with my pregnancies or with conceiving. However, I will admit that raising a child—or two, or three, or four—is quite literally the most challenging thing you will ever do, however it happens. Children are all so different. They listen differently, they learn differently, they cope differently. They are the most rewarding and most genuine creatures, too. They carry such innocence, and the only thing I know for sure is that I need to provide a life of stability for them; a life that I can dream of, where they never cross paths with some of the things that I did. I hope I can teach them a constructive and practical approach on how to treat people. I will do my absolute best to always make them feel deserving to have whatever they work hard enough for. I insist on showing them how to never doubt their worth, and that only they can decide who they are—no one else.

So, this is my hard stuff. This is what my vulnerability looks like. The truth is, I have never been someone who admits that she breaks down and falls apart. I never wanted people to know that they were influencing me or had a hold on me. Maybe the real problem for me was I felt that if I showed that I had this weakness and that it was taking over, it might open the door to how often it was actually happening. The growth we take on as human beings is OUR choice. We get to choose what happens; we get to choose to take control. I spent so much time being tough on the outside, when deep down I was deteriorating and had never felt more alone.

The important part for me was realizing that I was enough... AS I WAS. So let me tell you: YOU ARE ENOUGH, AS YOU ARE. You have the right to your emotions, and you have the right to navigate them however you feel benefits you best. If someone else is struggling in a similar area, it is likely that your coping strategies are different and it doesn't have to take away from you and your feelings.

We need to learn how to be more supportive of one another. I have come across some pretty amazing people in my life. Some I miss incredibly, some have taught me things, some have brought laughter and good times, and others have brought tears and heartache. Some I can say with confidence that we parted because we likely would not have brought the best out of each other. For those people who made me realize what was most important and confirmed that what I looked like didn't have to have any bearing on what I could offer, thank you. I no longer need to be the person struggling with self-worth, struggling with building relationships, or struggling with acceptance. These things are hard to admit to ourselves sometimes, so I think it's important to acknowledge that they exist. I feel so blessed that I was saved from a very dark place. It is a place that I still struggle with from time to time, but I know that I am strong, courageous, bold, loving, and truthful. If I have confidence in myself, then I can exude confidence in my life. I have learned a lot, and I will continue to grow through this journey. Nothing is as it once was, and maybe that is just how it is intended to be.

Chapter 4
CHLOE-JEAN SUMMERS

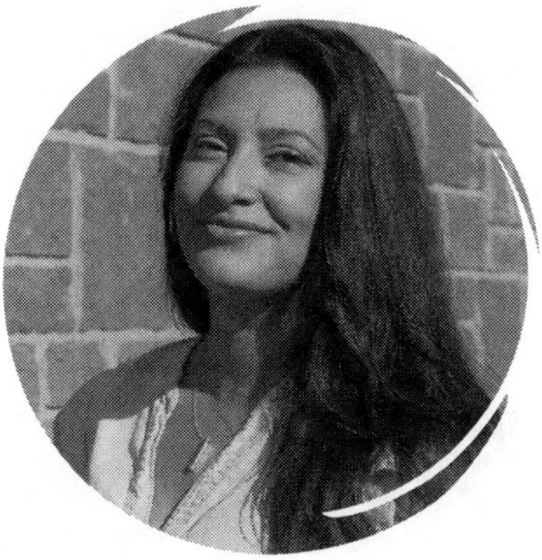

@chloejeansummers
chloejeansummers@outlook.com

Ok, I'm not saying Mondays are great or anything, but in my world they don't compare to the way Wednesdays can turn me into a straight up Jekyll and Hyde situation. Wednesdays in my house have been known to cause meltdowns, blowups, major potty mouth, and even timeouts. And I'm not talking about any of my three kids! It's all me, and it's all because every Wednesday for the past six years, my mother comes over to our house to help with the kids.

Now, before you assume that I'm ungrateful, let me explain. The relationship that I have with my mother has had major ups and downs. I mean, total bipolar waves. We've travelled to Europe, enjoyed some fabulously exquisite meals together, and shared our most deep and top-secret personal stories. We've also pushed each other, thrown things, used language that is downright disrespectful and ignorant, and I've even threatened that she would never see her second grandchild once he was born.

If I told you I was an only child would that make more sense to you? Maybe, maybe not. Are all girls like this with their moms, especially so when they have children of their own? Maybe, but maybe not. Is it because she's an Aquarius and I'm a Gemini? Who's in retrograde anyway? I can't keep track. Trust me, I've analyzed this issue for the past six years, found my way through the chaos and out onto the other side, and I have to tell you, it's LOVELY here! I went from self-medicating with alcohol, to CBD oil, therapy, and now I'm on prescription anti-anxiety SSRI medication and finally feeling content. I'm not saying my mother is the reason that I'm on meds now, but I can tell you that I went through hell and back analyzing our relationship to assess where and when we took a wrong turn, and I'm so grateful for where it's brought me.

I spent 25 years being the most positive, outgoing, smiley, and bubbly girl you'd ever meet. And honestly, I still am all of those things. But behind the scenes, and known to many of my close friends, I have battled with some challenges that I hide well and disclose to few. The biggest one is that my biological father isn't in my life and never has been. That is a chapter for another book, or maybe an entire book in itself. I did, however, have an incredible dad named Charlie who came into my life when I was about six months old and raised me like his own alongside my mom, Charlene. Now, at first glance, you might think, *okay so she's got "Daddy Issues"* but sadly, I'm going to get pretty candid about how I actually have some major mommy issues!

Before I can explain HOW this story has a heartwarming ending, I have to disclose now that it does, and that my mother was the first person to read this chapter. My hope is that through sharing my story about the relationship challenges that we've overcome, it will encourage hope in others facing similar challenges. There have been too many times that I've complained to friends and had them not only agree, but explain stories and frustrations with their own mothers. Sometimes when people tell you stories to try and relate to you, it makes you feel only partially less alone. For me, it was easier to laugh it off and send funny memes to friends than to really show how much my heart was breaking.

So let me paint a picture for you. It's Tuesday evening around 8pm. All three kids have been scrubbed clean of sidewalk chalk, Goldfish crackers, and sunscreen. They are snuggled into their beds and are giddy with excitement when they realize that Granny will be arriving in the morning. Santa should be jealous. The dishes are put away and there really isn't anything left to do but kick my feet up with Luke and relax. So we do! We pour a glass of wine, stare at our phones for longer than we should, and get caught up on all the social media nonsense that we missed during the day. And then it hits me. Tomorrow is Wednesday. WEDNESDAY!

Now my mouth gets dry as if I've just chugged this entire bottle of red and maybe choked down a spoonful of sawdust to top it off. My heart is racing. Why is my heart racing?! Is this wine caffeinated? When did I have my last sip of that coffee earlier? Do I have a heart issue? Is it getting worse?! I want to yell at Luke. I'm not quite sure why but my blood is boiling and I'm ready to rage.

He looks up from his phone. He's calm but cautious, probably because we do this every week. He starts to talk me down before I can even get a word out. My mother hasn't changed in 30 years. She's the same woman who packed my little kindergarten bento box lunches and pushed me in swing-sets...what IS MY

ISSUE?! Everything he's saying is true. Nothing about my mom has changed—if anything, she has done leaps and bounds to improve herself in every aspect of her life! She's sober, an avid reader, very into self-reflection and personal growth, and lord knows she helps us a substantial amount in the way of child care. But for some reason the anticipation of her arrival leaves me completely anxiety-ridden and quite heated.

I remember calling my dad and crying out of frustration that I couldn't just have a normal relationship with my mom. My parents separated when I was about 13 and it was incredibly amicable. So you can imagine he has nothing but kindness toward her and hates to see us not getting along in this way. He encouraged me to be more patient and sometimes would just listen to me cry and blubber on the phone. I know those conversations broke his heart, and it makes me sad to even write about it. But I feel like he was the best person to understand my frustrations, as he was married to her and would know her just as well as I do. Sadly, he couldn't wrap his head around it either. It's not that we have clashing personalities or that she somehow traumatized me in my youth. I just developed a severe anger toward her and it was progressively getting worse. My dad had the same kind of advice as Luke, and had promised that I would see my way through it.

So my mom has set out for the hour-long drive to our house every Wednesday to help minimize daycare costs and to spend some quality time with the grandkids ever since we had our first daughter. I am so thankful for all of the effort she puts in and the relationship that she's been able to build with all three of our kids. She never shows up empty-handed, either. She's always got a bag full of treats, new clothes for the kids in whatever character, favourite colour, or emoji they're into at the time, ingredients to help with dinner, a new magazine or notebook for me, and a big heart. But somewhere through all of this warm and fuzzy stuff that grandparents are made of, I see red. I get anxious thinking about the fights we're going to have for the next 24 hours or how awkward it's going to be at the dinner table if our fight was an afternoon session. I'm frustrated with her walk, her talk, her glance... everything about her sets me off. It wasn't always this bad, but the entire year of 2020 that coincided with a pandemic and my third and final maternity leave was the ultimate battle for me.

There were, of course, many reasons to feel overwhelmed and frustrated during the lockdown. At first, Luke and I put a little band-aid fix on my "Wednesday Scaries" by making margaritas, or just taking a random shot of tequila to try and minimize the tension. Then I tried taking CBD oil, which left me feeling warm and fuzzy but not quite as energetic as I need to be when there's a house full of toddlers.

There were Tuesday evenings when I would get into my comfiest clothes, get under my duvet, and curl up with the blanket up to my eyes trying to breathe slowly and deeply to calm my nerves in anticipation of spending an entire Wednesday with my mom. One time Luke even brought the CBD oil to me in bed and put a few drops on my tongue for me as I was on the edge of having a full-blown panic attack. I knew this wasn't a long-term solution, but approaching my mom with the idea of "mother-daughter therapy" was a long shot, and I wasn't ready for it to deteriorate our relationship any further.

The last big fight I remember having with my mom was on a Wednesday morning within five minutes of her arrival. She walked in and I don't remember what was said, but I know that I was on edge because of her arrival and I said something that instigated an argument. Luke and I were going out that day to do a Costco run and various other errands while she graciously hung out with the kids.

So Luke was getting dressed, starting the car, and ready to walk out the door when I was just getting into a screaming match with my mom in the front entranceway. Honestly, she hadn't even had a minute to remove her shoes. With one last fiery exit statement, I stormed out of the house and into the truck where we drove silently for most of the 45-minute ride to Costco. At some point I was crying, and Luke just turned down the music and put his hand on my hand. It's in these moments when I'm so grateful for him, but at the same time just utterly confused as to why his mom could raise him to be such a courteous and calm human being and I'm, well... the way that I am! I drive myself nuts with my own behaviour and reactions.

I cried in Costco and I cried on the way home. It was awful. I guess it was probably my breaking point. That day, instead of happily anticipating the latest and greatest snacks in store for us, I'd played out all of the recent mother/daughter fights in my head and continuously analyzed them. Why does it stress me out to have her here? She is SO helpful, and loving, and warm, and the kids adore her! Luke is right when he tells me, "she's the same mom you've always had; nothing has changed." That is true! So why do I get SO incredibly angry with her and toward her? I wish I didn't spew those awful words at her. She doesn't deserve that, and *I* wouldn't forgive me for it.

I spent a few years telling close friends that I think I would benefit from doing therapy sessions with my mom. The only issue is trying to approach my mother about this idea and the potential of it totally ruining our relationship. That would be an absolute nightmare and the risk was too high. So I ended up deciding it wasn't the right choice, or at least not the right time. Instead, I signed up for a free Cognitive Behaviour Therapy workshop that had popped up on my Instagram feed. (Okay, sometimes it benefits us to have our phones listening to us.) It was hosted by McMaster University and was free, as it was part of the graduate research program about postpartum depression. It was one full eight-hour day online, with a group of 29 other moms led by the head of the Psychology Department there.

During the workshop, we learned about Cognitive Behaviour Therapy and how it can benefit postpartum mothers—and also anyone, in any situation, really—who is looking to dig a bit deeper into their issues and find their way to the surface! Almost all of us were suffering with different problems, and it was refreshing to know that I wasn't alone in taking these foreign feelings so hard. The positive side to over-analyzing things in your life is that you're actively looking for change. Sometimes there's so much that goes on in our heads, and as mothers, there typically isn't any time to take care of our mental well-being. We can't even pee by ourselves, let alone sit with our thoughts and find reasonable solutions. A LOT gets swept under the rug when you enter into motherhood and your "self" becomes a low priority.

So at one point in the workshop we took turns telling stories about things that trigger us and where our outbursts, frustrations, or fears come from. I took this time to reflect on my biggest issue, which was how motherhood had somehow rocked my relationship with my mother. Yes, being a mom is hard and it doesn't matter if you are a first, second, or third-time mom. But I was ready for the body image adjustments, the midnight cluster feeding, the zombie eyes, and permanent mom-bun. I have an incredibly supportive partner in this and we balance each other in our parenting. It's been a learning process, believe me, but it's been a positive one. What I wasn't ready for was the resentment and rage that I would feel for my own mother.

What I realized from the CBT therapy was that I have the power to choose how things make me feel. Even if something is directed toward me out of frustration or anger, I have the ability to choose whether to let it affect me or not.

Growing up and becoming an adult makes you realize and appreciate that your parents are just people at the end of the day. They were kids who grew up. They made choices along the way that weren't always the best ones, but ultimately they led to you being on this planet, and THAT is something to be grateful for. Their mistakes or wrong turns weren't wrong turns at all. Everything they ever said or did, every relationship—good or bad—all led to them having you, their greatest accomplishment. Only YOU can choose how something makes you feel. If that doesn't empower you, I don't know what will!

This is just a different approach to how I have been handling a lot of relationships in my life. I am naturally quite sensitive and take things critically (cue the childhood piano lessons and art classes). That's my personality and I'm not trying to be someone different. I'm working on taking things in stride, putting perspective on conversations or wording, and developing resilience and confidence in my own choices, overall. I'm realizing that just because I was parented in a certain way, I can now choose which aspects of my upbringing I'm going to put into my own parenting style, and which will be left in the past. The same ideas and virtues that served my parents may or may not work for me, and I won't know for sure until I test them out. It's just funny how things can trigger you and catch you off guard so dramatically!

One that stands out for me is a memory from grade school. I was probably around grade 2 or 3, and we lived so close to the school that my mom would walk over to pick me up for lunch most days. But one day, she didn't show up! This is long before the days of needing to be signed out or picked up at the office. So I was standing outside by the gate waiting as the other kids who went home for lunch all left with their parents. Even then, I knew she didn't just forget about me—I am an only child after all. I was her ONLY priority—zero competing and zero sharing to be had! My nerves were at an all-time high even for anxious little me. So, I racked my brain. *What would my mom want me to do right now? Should I go inside and cry to a teacher or just walk home? I'm sure I can handle it. We know the crossing guard by first name and her kids go to my school as well. I even know a few people who live on the streets that lead me home, should anything happen and I need help.* So I chose in that moment to trek home alone. I wasn't scared, but I definitely walked a little faster than normal and was wondering the whole time if my mom would be happily waiting for my arrival. When I went in she was working on a client (she ran her own aesthetics business out of our home), and she had a huge smile on her face and said something to the effect of "you did it! You walked home all by yourself! I knew you would figure it out, how was that?" And I guess at that age, and with my sensitive personality, I was quite confused. Here I am, scared and alone, and she's proud of me?

Fast forward now about 25 years later, and here I was late picking our oldest daughter up from preschool. She was the last kid there just standing with the teacher holding hands. She wasn't upset but just seemed confused and worried. But the guilt that I felt for months—even years—after that could have eaten me alive. It reminded me of that one time from my childhood... ONE TIME!!

Being on the parenting side of this situation made me frustrated with myself, not with my parents. I shouldn't have been late. Now, does our daughter even remember this incident? Probably not, as she was only three years old. But it'll stay with *me* and has already made me more punctual for school and daycare.

Learning to be gentle with myself is something that I've really put a focus on while on my final maternity leave during a pandemic. If we have Kraft Dinner twice in one week, the kids are pumped and it makes my life a heck of a lot easier. So taking this perspective with my own parents and their experience raising me has given me a lot of peace. We're all here doing the best we can and sometimes it's really freakin' hard!

I think with anger, it's easier to deflect it onto someone or something else and push it out of your head as much as possible. It's very easy to judge other people for just about anything, and it's funny (not actually funny, but interesting) that we seem to vividly remember all of the times that we were hard done by, or rejected, or not picked. And yet, there is an abundance of positivity in our life that we so easily forget and leave in the past.

After I completed the CBT workshop, there were follow up emails and questionnaires to check on our progress. They wanted to see if we were putting it into our daily or even weekly use, and if it was benefitting us at all. For me it has kick started an 18-month (and growing) personal growth mission. The positive changes in my life happened so quickly when I took control of my own feelings and decided to be less affected by the negative—and more appreciative for the positive.

I grew up Roman Catholic and developed my own sense of spirituality as an adult that has led me through tons of researching to find what kind of faith best serves me. I have always been fascinated with Buddhism and the focus on letting go of the ego and being present. I don't think it really matters what religion or faith you follow to appreciate those two concepts. So I read books on meditation, Buddhism, spirituality, parenting, psychology, and the odd fiction paperback in between to ease the heaviness of some of this info.

I decided that I wasn't going to waste my final maternity leave crying, being angry, resentful, ruining relationships, and building crappy memories for my children. What a waste of time! My motto was, "I'm going to work on myself. That's the only thing I can change, and if I'm the best version of me I will be able to handle anything. When I'm the best that I can be, everything else will come naturally." And I can tell you that it's quite the powerful statement to tell yourself daily, sometimes hourly!

I started listening to guided meditations and I would just lay on my bed and cry through them. It was incredibly freeing and felt like a little cleanse every time. Eventually I didn't cry through them anymore and could focus on my breath. Then I started to go for walks, at first by myself and then my neighbourhood friends would suggest that we go together, which was so much more fun! At one point I had a different walking buddy for every day of the week and it was 45 - 60 minutes that we could sweat it out and belly laugh our way around the block.

I chose to be forgiving with myself. This translates into many areas of my life, but a few that stand out are in the kitchen and with household chores. If meals are balanced and everyone likes them... who am I kidding, that never happens! And as far as household chores go, if it was a nice day, we would spend it outside swimming, going to the park, and getting ice cream. If the laundry stays in the basket for the week, no big deal! I don't step on the scale every day. I eat chocolate when and how often I need to, and I nurture friendships that bring me joy.

The way that I took this new attitude toward my relationship with my mom has been the ultimate success story. I learned to listen more and speak less. If you met me you'd know how hard that is—I quite literally don't stop talking! Even though it's challenging for me, I find that I now have time to hear what people are really saying. I have time to acknowledge how things make them feel and to see that maybe I need to spend more time nurturing our relationship. I started listening to the things my mom would say to me, and even when some things came off a touch passive-aggressive, I can make light of it—and we can actually joke about it now. And instead of muttering awful names under my breath in the other room or when I close the door to send my mom home for the night, we jokingly say, "oh Granny Bananny" and we all laugh. Sometimes we belly laugh now at the things that used to send me off on a tangent and have me slamming the dishwasher door shut and crying in the bathroom.

Being open and honest with her has helped as well. We take time when the kids go to bed or they're playing nicely in the toy room to chat, and although it's not typically serious conversations, we can bring things up openly and honestly and get to the root of them on the spot. I sit and watch in awe as she reads to our youngest daughter and teaches her new words and songs. The kids are so good for her. They do some things so obediently for her that I could never get them to do for me!

Going through mental health struggles during the pandemic is a common thread, and I hope that everyone can have a success story through to the other wonderful side that is contentment. I can tell you that working on yourself, staying grounded, being thankful, and waking up with a gracious heart every day is a great start. I've learned to appreciate every moment with every person I choose to surround myself with. And after spending so much time with myself on lockdown, I really had time to think about who I want to spend my time with.

My mom has been an absolute angel through all of this. She's had struggles of her own, and has picked herself back up and brushed herself off time and time again. That's just one of her most admirable qualities. She's the hardest working woman

I've ever met. Her warm energy radiates off of her, she fills a room with laughter and love, and you are blessed to be a part of her life. I'm incredibly thankful that she was so open and loving through all of the crap that I put her through, but then again, that says a lot about her heart.

We hug a little harder, we laugh louder, and I miss her so much when she leaves now. I can't even go to bed when she's here unless we've hugged it out—like really hugged it out! The focus I've put on bettering our relationship has benefitted us in ways I never thought possible. I'm so proud of us. I want this for everyone who struggles with their relationships with their own parents or family members.

You can do this. Not every story in this book will resonate with you, but if this one does, my hope is that you can see the light at the end of our story and try to gain some perspective into your own situation. Who knows, maybe you'll get your happy ending and be booking a retreat with YOUR mom—and writing a wonderful chapter in a book someday, too. And if so, I can't wait to read it. Life is my personal growth journey, and I plan on making the most of every moment. I hope you do too!

Chapter 5
DANIELLE LEHMKUHL

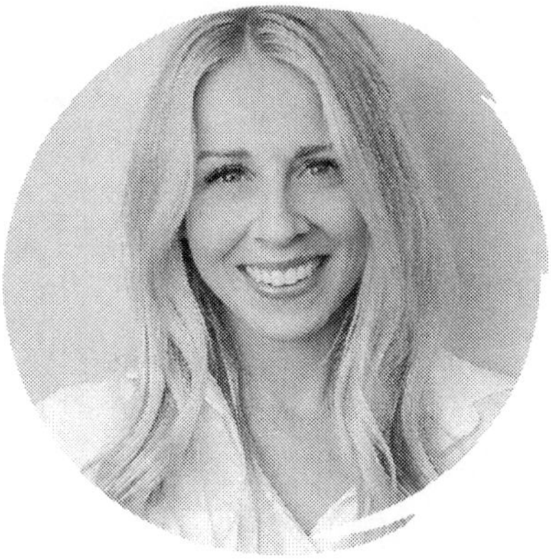

@be.naturelle

Disclaimer: I understand that my thoughts and feelings may be triggers for some. These triggers may bring up feelings of distaste, resentment, and hostility toward my words and me as a human being. My situation was a trigger that I had to learn to navigate and cope with. I acknowledge that situations in my life that I struggled with may be situations that some are praying for. I honour those people and send support and love to those who hope to bring life into this world, and who hope to be parents one day. I hope that throughout this chapter, individuals see that I had these thoughts toward my experiences because of external pressure and expectations, not because of my internal beliefs and values.

7:00 a.m. — October 12:

The very moment and day that changed everything. The day that has led me to honouring my true self and the day that I am *now* forever grateful for. I say "now" because these thoughts and feelings did not come easily. Although it has been an emotional and whirlwind of a journey, I can now say that I am appreciative of these experiences, as they have led me to living a life filled with self-compassion, self-acceptance, and, might I mention, one powerful, exhilarating, and badass attitude of *you either accept me or carry on in life without me.* I understand that statement can come with perceptions that I have an "I don't give a fuck" attitude, but that's not the case. I care about a lot, but what I mean by that is that I no longer hold space in my life for people, things, or experiences that don't serve me and/or don't embrace who I am, my decisions, my journey, and my choices. This is not me rebelling against the world; this is me confidently showing up in this world as the person I am designed to be and the person that I deserve to be, and let's face it—I think my choices and decisions in life have made me turn out... not so bad.

Throughout this chapter, I express my thoughts and feelings on my life. At no point am I here to say that any other sequence of events in someone else's life is wrong, as I believe there is no "wrong." Your thoughts, your feelings, your emotions, and your experiences are yours. Own the shit out of them. Everyone is different, and no two people experience life the same way, just as no two people are the same—and that, my friend, is a beautiful thing.

My childhood was more than I could have asked for. I was blessed with loving parents, a loving sister, and I was provided for beyond my wildest dreams. My parents divorced when I was young, so the memories of a traditional family of four are sparse and limited. However, despite the separation, my parents filled our lives with love, wonderful co-parenting, values, and direction in life.

I always felt in life that I wanted to be someone different. I wanted to go against the grain—well, so it felt. At the time, it may have been perceived as rebellion, when really, it truly was me being pulled into alignment. Alignment is when your body, mind, soul, and spirit are operating in the way they should. You create energy and you feel that energy—energy that is powerful and desirable. I did not want to follow society's plan, but it was portrayed that steering away from that plan was a rebellious or defiant act. I dreamed of picking up and moving away, but that was seen as irresponsible. I desired self-expression, but I was conditioned into thinking that it was "unladylike" or "rough" looking. I yearned for something greater than the nine-to-five, but I was influenced into thinking that a pension represented freedom and success. So, like many, I existed. I existed in this life going through the motions and I sure as hell didn't ever question those motions. I didn't honour those feelings and desires, and that is what led me to several moments of suffering and lack of confidence in my true identity.

From a young age, society, parenting, educational systems, and the media have instilled this hierarchy-based approach to life. You go to school, and you go to school because you need to BE someone. Your goal at the end of all of this schooling is to establish a career—to define the "who" you are in life—well, so we are told. Something I've noticed along this journey is that oftentimes if you've never met someone before, the second or third question they may ask you after asking your name is, "What do you do?" "What are you?" These questions consistently condition the mind into thinking that the WHO they are is really associated with WHAT they do—what they label themselves, whether it be a teacher, a business employee, a manager—you name it. There is nothing wrong in associating yourself with what you do for your career, but I want you to really dig deep into knowing WHO you truly are, minus the job that you do. Challenge yourself in knowing the who, embracing the who, and honouring the who, because in finding all of that, comes a life filled with joy, alignment, and ease.

Tip #1: Get rid of all of the titles. Take them all away and ask yourself, "Who am I?" What are the greatest things you exemplify and what brings you passion?

Following a career comes buying a car, buying a house, finding a partner, getting engaged, getting married, and, of course, having children. These are the hierarchical steps in life that will lead you to "happiness," or so they say..."They" being these unwritten rules that you must follow in order to achieve "The American Dream" or, shall I say, "The Canadian Dream"...Eh?

Rightfully so, I lived life with these expectations that I would follow through and achieve these big milestones. I believe the world to be very linear and set up so that you achieve and work toward "accomplishments" in order to receive a sense of recognition or purpose. But why? Why can't we just focus on recognizing each other's happiness and existence? That's what we need to focus on.

I obtained a degree, landed a career, bought a car, bought a house, found a partner, and... surprise, had a baby... no big deal. Well that's a lie; it *was* a big deal for me. The pregnancy was an experience in life that brought me from my lowest lows to now being a reason that has lifted me up beyond what I could have ever imagined.

Despite this transformation being the reason for a lot of heartache and tears, it is a change that I now believe that I needed. It was a change that was meant to be in order to become aligned with who and where I am today. Let's just say amen to that.

The two pink lines. They were the beginning of a forever and the beginning of an internal shift that was about to happen, but also the beginning of a whole lot of "What the actual fuck?"

moments. The thoughts began to spiral:

"I can't have a child right now."

"Oh boy, what are my parents going to think of me? I'm not married!"

"I have failed."

"What are others going to think of me?"

"Should I be going through with this?"

I began my pregnancy in shame—shame that I was not married, that I did not follow through with life as to how it was expected of me and how it *should* be. *Should* is a word that I have felt deeply. I *should* do this and I *should* do that. I have left the word "should" in the hands of others—their opinions, their thoughts—when all along, *should* is something that we as human beings SHOULD hold onto for ourselves. That comes with not allowing the "shoulds" to be in possession of others, but to be in possession of yourself. The shoulds need to be your desires, your beliefs, and your actions that feel aligned with you.

I began to share the news with the people in my life. I had to, because at the end of the day, this was happening. I shared the news and consistently followed up with the explanations. I would acknowledge the fact that I was not married, and that I did not plan this for my life at this point. I felt overwhelmed every time I had to tell another person because I knew I was opening up the opportunity for me to be judged and for my "thoughts" about this situation to become reality.

At times, it became reality. I was consistently asked if this was a planned pregnancy and it was consistently assumed that I was a married woman. Moments like these are ones that forced me to dig deeper into the origin of those assumptions and questions and to really challenge the meaning of them as a human being. At times, it led me to a place of confidence in knowing that my life was absolutely valuable, despite the curves and, at other times, it put me back into feelings of shame and failure.

I remember speaking with my doctor when I was a few weeks along. He knew the struggles that I was having and said something that began to shift my perspective in all of this. He said, "Danielle, you know it's 2020, right?" It was a question so simple, yet so powerful. I left that day and really started to replay that comment in my mind and challenge the thoughts that I was having inside my head. I kept thinking "Yeah!! It's 2020... new era, new realities, new life plans. University wasn't as common 50 years ago, first-time home buyers were buying homes for $500,000, not all people were placing marriage on this high pedestal anymore." Things were different and that was okay.

So why didn't I *feel* okay? I know for a fact that had I received this news after being married and intentionally planning this, I would have felt completely different. I would have seen this as a celebration, yet I let external expectations dictate my thoughts and feelings of a situation. I have missed out on moments and experiences that I will never have again because I let these conditioned beliefs get the best of me. I recognized this, and that is when I started to begin the journey of accepting my life as it was, how it will be, and how it has played out.

"I started to begin the journey of accepting my life as it was, how it will be, and how it has played out."

This sentence is one that I changed. As I sit here with my thoughts, I automatically wrote "This is when I *accepted* my life as it was, how it will be, and how it has played out" and I realized that's not true. I recognized the thought, challenged the thought, worried about expressing my true feelings, and shifted my feelings into a place of acceptance. It was automatic for me to write "accepted" but to me that word represents completion—fully, 100 percent, completely taking hold of that "thing" (life)—and that is definitely not something that I have achieved yet, and may never will. What I do know, however, is that I embrace life fully—100 percent and completely.

I bring this to light because I acknowledge that this is still a journey. I am not perfect. I have not accomplished everything in my life that I wish to, whether that be the act of doing, thinking, healing, growing, or shifting. I still go through waves, as most of us do, and I have good days and bad days. However, the fact that I have more good days than not, and more acceptance than resistance, is what keeps me continuing to push through.

As I battled with my feelings toward the pregnancy, I began to notice little victories. Although they were small, they kept me going. I continued to place importance on the value of my thoughts and challenged the inner critic when it arose. When I express my thoughts and feelings of where I am now and my current awareness of conditioning, it comes from a place of hard work and time. I can confidently say that I did not have a lot of these realizations during my pregnancy, but it's because of the pregnancy and events that occurred during it that sparked this state of reflection on my thoughts and feelings.

I began to find joy in the experience and focused my attention on the exciting moments: the ultrasounds, the kicks and movement, the gender reveal, the baby shower, and getting the nursery ready. Might I mention that this pregnancy was during a time of uncertainty, anxiety, despair, and tragedy—the COVID-19 pandemic. This was a time when I was not able to share moments with family like I wanted to. I was not able to have my partner, Adam, with me during my checkups. He wasn't able to hear the heartbeat in real time. I spent days isolated to protect myself and the baby, and I was limited to purchasing all of the exciting baby items online.

As feelings of shame and failure arose surrounding my inability to “achieve societal expectations,” I acknowledged that these feelings were there because of conditioning, not because I truly believed them to be true. I knew that it was okay. I knew that I could love and support the child. I knew the child came from a place of love, and I knew that this baby was going to have unconditional love from everyone. With these realizations, I tried to focus on the things that mattered to ME… shocking! Here I was starting to put my thoughts and opinions first, not others.

Tip #2: Identify your beliefs and desires, let go of the external pressures and opinions, and learn to embrace and support your beliefs and desires.

Throughout the pregnancy there were many decisions to be made. With these decisions, I saw the opportunity for me to take back my power, control of my thoughts, and, essentially, my life. One of the first decisions that I faced was choosing to have an obstetrician or a midwife. Being someone that was rooted in choosing a more holistic approach to life (yes, the “woo woo-eyeroll-weirdo” kind of things), I chose a midwife. I knew that if I ever experienced a birth, I hoped for it to be one including a midwife with natural remedies and support in order to deliver the baby. I felt good about that decision, but, once again, being surrounded with very right-winged opinions, it turned into me explaining the “whys” and essentially defending my decisions. When worries would arise, I aimed to remember that this was MY decision, MY choice, and MY birth plan.

With a very supportive midwife team and an extremely supportive partner, I was looking forward to the birth and to the moment that I was going to meet my son for the first time.

While I looked into the future, I saw these amazing moments of pure happiness, joy, and love, embracing the state of being in those first few moments. This perception is all I knew. I was told that at that moment of birth it's essentially butterflies and rainbows. Who wouldn't want to experience that?

So, as I approached my due date—amidst a full kitchen renovation and lockdown—I was looking forward to having time to rest and enjoy the last few weeks of carrying this miracle.

Thanksgiving 2020 was a day that had been planned to be a slow start—enjoying a coffee in the morning, sending condolences via Zoom for a loved one's funeral, and finishing with a small dinner to celebrate all that we were thankful for... especially the baby that was set to be arriving in four-and-a-half weeks.

Well, that plan was taken away from me. It was one of the many plans throughout this journey that was taken away.

It was 7:00 a.m. on October 12th. I was laying there thinking, "What the hell?! Danielle... Did you just lose control of your bladder?" I launched out of bed, waddled over to the bathroom, and experienced a feeling I most definitely had never felt before. The taps were on and holy moly... my water broke. But how? I still had 4.5 weeks left! I had no bags packed and I had not really prepared for this day as I thought I had some time to get there. Within seconds, the cramping I had been experiencing for the last three days really ramped up and I thought *Oh, wow! These are what contractions feel like!!* All of the thoughts went through my mind within minutes. I knew the baby was breech at the last ultrasound and there I was hoping that he had turned head down, because as we all know, I wanted a smooth delivery with my midwives. If the baby was breech, that meant I would need a cesarean section.

There we were, throwing whatever we could grab into the suitcase, managing the chaos, the dogs, getting the baby bag packed and heading out to the hospital. Within thirty minutes my life went from a relaxing day thinking about the next 4.5 weeks of the baby and I being one unit—to having contractions a minute-and-a-half apart, with broken water, heading to the hospital.

To some, this is a possibility that would be easily managed. To me, it was a moment that changed everything. The shock, the numbness, the "grey" memories—everything changed.

Getting into the car and heading to the hospital is where the memories begin to fade and seeing this written out today still carries so much hurt, pain, and suffering. I remember going to the hospital, and not once did I really realize that the baby was most likely going to be there within hours. I don't remember what I thought, and I sure as hell know what I felt—contractions—but I don't remember mentally how I was feeling. When the nurses realized how fast the contractions were progressing, we were told, "You're having the baby today!"

It still feels like such a blur. The best way I can describe it is that it feels grey. It's not clear and I don't have vivid memories of my feelings, but I now recognize that I was in complete shock as to what was occurring. When they confirmed that the baby was still breech, I realized that I had lost all control of everything I had planned. Although my midwives were with me, this was not what we had hoped and planned for. This is when the extreme shock factor kicked in. This is when being "present" in the moment was completely taken away from me and the "what the fuck?" factor took over and dictated the hours of several days, weeks, and months of my life to follow.

Within minutes I was hooked up, poked, prepped, and laying

on the emergency room table with what felt like a busy downtown street of doctors and nurses buzzing around me. Adam came into the room and I thought he would offer me comfort and clarity in the reality of it all, but when I looked back at him I realized that he, too, was experiencing the "what the fuck?" factor just like I was. There were no moments of "Okay, let's do this!" or "This is so exciting!" or "Aren't you excited to meet our baby boy?" This is where I struggled the most, because I began to panic due to the fact that I was not feeling what everyone told me I would feel. I felt numb and cold. Quite frankly, I felt nothing. I was too overwhelmed with the shock to really be present in the moment and enjoy what was about to happen.

At 11:06, out came our baby boy, crying and seemingly healthy to the doctor's eyes. Here it came—the minute that I was about to see my baby for the first time. The magical moment was about to arrive. A few minutes later, there he was, and although I felt emotion, it was not the emotion that I had expected. I realize that I felt that way because of the shock and chaos that took place on that day, but it doesn't make it easier that I still don't truly remember the feeling of seeing my child for the first time. My body was consumed with confusion and shock. I would do anything to have that moment over again, to be able to really embrace the firsts, but I never will. I continue to focus on accepting and acknowledging that it is okay; there are many other firsts that I have and will experience. However, it does not make the pain of missing the very first seem any easier.

Tip #3: Focus on shifting your mindset. Acknowledge the pain and suffering and shift your perspective into one of positivity. I lost the memories of the first look, but I shifted the perspective into knowing that I will have many other important "firsts."

Again, this created another feeling of failure, because I did not *feel* the way that society had told me and expected me to *feel.* I realize that my feelings and experiences on that day were real, hard, traumatizing, and, most importantly, out of my control. I now allow myself to have self-compassion over that event and give myself grace in feeling the emotions that are associated with an emergency, out of the blue, early, and quick cesarean section. Throughout this journey I have taken these signs and moments of remembrance to really honour the progress and growth that I have made as a human being, because let's face it: life can be hard and it's all about working through the hard shit in order to live a life full of abundance and ease.

Tip #4: Honour your feelings as true and valuable. Don't set your expectations based on the outer world. Focus on being present with YOUR feelings and YOUR emotions, as they are yours and no one else's.

Like the birth experience, I imagined the first moments of holding my son to be ones that overwhelmed me with happiness and joy. However, with major bleeding and priorities of my health being at the forefront, I did not have this magical moment. I know I eventually held him, but my emotions and memories are sparse and blurred. Looking back I remember the infamous words, "It could be worse," and at no point do I believe that statement to be false. What I have learned, however, is that it is so important to accept that just because there may be worse in the world, it does not mean that any person's "worse" is less than someone else's.

After a few days in the hospital, we were sent home. It was a surreal experience, to say the least. Here we were: two parents, being sent into this world to care for, raise, and protect this tiny little bundle of joy that we had created.

I left the hospital with expectations that once again, life was going to be happy and exciting. I knew that I was struggling with the way things had played out, but I assumed that the next few days, weeks, and months would outweigh all of those struggles.

As the days progressed, I had all the emotional waves that I now know to be quite "normal." In those moments, however, I had no realization that this was, for the most part, expected post-birth feelings. The thing that I struggled with is that no one told me about the downs and the overwhelming emotions. Everyone just talked about the good things; yet, at times, I didn't know what those good things were. I remember saying numerous times, "I don't feel happy," "I feel really sad," and "I don't feel good." I had just dealt with an internal battle of allowing myself to feel positive about this pregnancy. I had just unexpectedly had my baby four-and-a-half weeks early. I had had some serious complications post birth, and now I was facing one of my biggest uphill battles.

Postpartum.

Physically, you are dealing with healing. Mentally, you are dealing with exhaustion. Emotionally, you are dealing with the hormones and experiences, yet it is a time when some expect you to be over the moon with how your life has become.

Although I look back and wish some things could have been different, I am "accepting" (again, it's a process and I haven't fully, 100 percent, completely gotten there) of how things worked out. I have taken time to grieve. Yes, I know it's an interesting choice of words. So many of us automatically associate "grief" with the loss of a loved one, but grief is present when someone feels a deep amount of sadness and suffering.

If there is one word that I would use to describe my overall feelings around the birth, it would be grief. I needed time—and still need time—to sit with my feelings surrounding the birth.

I'm grieving the loss of my birth plan, the loss of what I thought I would feel when I delivered my son, the loss of memories on that day that were blinded by shock, and the loss of my happiness that has taken a while to find. With that being said, however, I have grown and come to peace in accepting that I am worthy of feeling the way that I felt.

I say this because despite all of the struggles I have expressed, those struggles have led me to a place of understanding, growth, self-compassion, advocacy, and alignment—all of the things that I needed a little bit more of in my life.

I needed an understanding of trauma. No matter how small or big it may seem, trauma is trauma. Grief is grief, no matter what other people think; what matters is what you feel. I have grown beyond what I could have imagined and what I thought I needed. I have grown as an individual, a mother, a daughter, and a partner. I have grown my self-compassion for my journey, and for the journey of others. I have become one of strength and understanding of myself and others that experience similar thoughts and feelings, no matter what the catalysts of those feelings are. I have grown in my advocacy for traumatic births and postpartum. I support and honour all pregnancy and birth experiences, no matter what that looks like. I now have alignment with my true self and desires. I have found the world of human design and fully embraced the journey that it has taken me on to arrive here.

Life is not about putting pain and grief on a continuum. Life is about what "pain," "suffering," and "grief" are to that person in your life. What is THEIR struggle? What is THEIR story? And while learning that and honouring that, it is important to recognize that their story is not your story. Although many people may not perceive or understand why certain events cause pain and suffering, it is important to listen and understand with empathy. At the end of the day, everyone has had different experiences, different upbringings, different biological base lines, and different expectations as to how their life will come to plan.

I have grown. I have taken the hard times as an opportunity to allow myself to reflect internally in regard to the conditioning and opinions of others. I recognize that so many of us exist in this lifetime and operate in sequence—achieving, accomplishing, and succeeding. However, I have shifted from that paradigm and taken time to truly embrace who I am and what I desire—not what others desire—and to live each day in alignment with my true self. I have accepted that there is no wrong in my life because of my decisions, and as I live life from a place of love, support, and acceptance, that is a life that I can be proud of.

This major event in my life has taken me from a place of "stress when conformity is not obtained"—to bliss, acceptance, and individuality. I lost control over a lot of things in those almost nine months of carrying a baby and several months postpartum, all because I allowed external expectations and societal pressure to get the best of me. I lost control over my feelings, my thoughts, and my emotions because I let the feelings, thoughts, and emotions of others get the best of me. The loss of control that I experienced has blissfully led me to a place of power, acceptance, self-compassion, and absolute alignment. I embrace who I am designed to be. I embrace the path that life has led me down so far, and I embrace the feelings of alignment with truly being who I desire to be.

I have always said that you have one life. That's it. Yesterday is gone; the memories are there. Today is a present; make the best of it. Tomorrow is around the corner; take it as it comes. By allowing yourself to live a life in which you honour yourself—honouring your quirks, your desires, and your passions—

it guides you to a life of ease, in which you gain control of who you are truly meant to be.

Throughout this hard time I have grown and birthed an amazing son, experienced unconditional love from my partner, have had a supportive family, and I live a life honouring my true self and who I want to be. I have handled the hard stuff by challenging my thoughts and beliefs, and that has led me to a place of happiness and acceptance of my life today. I now am my most powerful and authentic self. I found growth and my true intentions within the challenges that I faced.

Tip #5: Be you. Make a life for yourself that follows your beliefs and desires. Be true to who you want to be and live life with passion.

Be authentic. Be an unapologetic version of your true self and handle it like a boss!

Chapter 6
DR. MANDY LEE

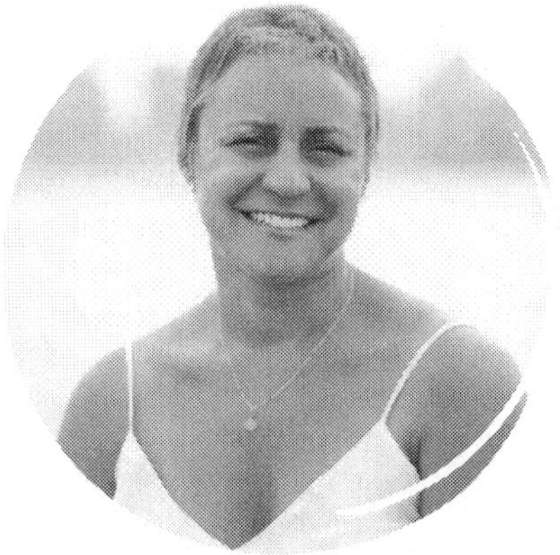

Photographer: Caitlin McCaulley/McCaulley Photograph

Instagram @drmandylee, Twitter @DrMandyLeeDC
www.drmandylee.com

I sat in the sterile waiting room of the ER listening to the beeps, alarms, and hushed voices of those sitting around me. I watched the nurses and doctors whiz by me, working in what seemed like perfectly organized chaos. I had never been to the ER before—EVER. In fact, I could count on one hand (okay... maybe two if you count the chronic ear aches I had as a child) the number of times I had been to see a doctor over my 39 years of life. I had been healthy my whole life; actually, ultra healthy—if that is even a thing. I rarely had a cold, never the flu, and no weird rashes to report. By all accounts, I did everything "right." I ate healthy food. I got enough sleep each night, and I dedicated my life to making others healthier. I was working full-time as a chiropractor and teaching multiple fitness classes a week as my side gig. I was tired but fulfilled. I was in love with my life and felt great satisfaction that every day I was making a difference. Then it ALL came to a screeching halt. I went from 100 to 0 all at once.

I waited in the ER that day for what seemed like an eternity. I called my office and asked my receptionist to reschedule my patients as things were a little slower than I expected at the hospital. The radiologist who had just read my ultrasound wanted me to make a "quick stop" afterwards to see the ER doc. I had been experiencing some vague symptoms in the past couple of months—a frequent need to pee at night (nocturia), some mild low back pain, a stuck feeling in my lower abdomen when I attempted up-dog in the yoga classes I was teaching, and, in **hindsight**, maybe a deeper fatigue than I usually felt. None of these things slowed me down though, so I was not worried. I continued to work hard, and I racked my brain and used my extensive medical knowledge to try and figure out what might be causing my issues. I suspected a bladder infection, yeast infection, or some other benign reason for how I was feeling. I was working out too much, working too hard, and not taking any time to relax or take care of myself. I would make changes to my schedule as I had promised myself not that long ago.

Finally, a nurse called my name, brought me into a private room, and told me that the doctor would be in soon. I sat there completely ignorant to the fact that my ENTIRE life was about to change in the next five minutes. I was sitting alone in that room, as I had not thought that it was necessary to bring someone for a quick investigative trip to get an ultrasound. The first question the doctor asked me was "Are you married?"

"Yes," I replied.

"Do you have kids?"

"No."

"How long have you had these symptoms?"

"A couple of months, maybe."

"Have you experienced any bloating or cramps?"

"Uhmm... when I eat gluten or dairy, so I avoid that," I told him. And then he dropped a literal bomb. He said that he didn't like what he saw on the ultrasound. I had a pelvic mass that measured a whopping 10 cm. This is why they had trouble visualizing one of my ovaries on the ultrasound; it had been pushed off to the side by this mass. I was listening intently to what he said, but not YET pushing the panic button. Everything I was hearing was swirling around in my head—pelvic mass, 10 cm, hidden ovary. My entire world came to a stop when he finished by saying..."These are the days I hate my job... here you are sitting in front of me looking so damn healthy, but I would be remiss if I did not tell you what it looks like: ovarian cancer."

I didn't say much after that, as I was at a total loss for words. If you know me, you know that this just does not happen. I sat there stunned, trying to comprehend every word that was just hurled in my direction. Cancer? Me? How? I sat waiting for my CT scan (which they ordered immediately to see if there were any other spots) and I looked down at my hands, visibly shaking, which was also something new. I considered myself rock solid; I had lived as a fierce, confident woman, able to handle life with ease and tackle any hardships life had thrown at me in the past. This, however, was a new ballgame, with no comparison to any trials and tribulations I had previously experienced. It quite literally left me shaking and brought me to my knees.

The rest of my stay in the hospital that day included a couple of phone calls to my mom (who lives in a different province), my husband (who was out of town at the time), and a call to my "work wife." She picked up the phone when I called and I said "It's bad. I need you to come here." She was crying before she even walked into the room. No tears fell from my eyes; that's what shock will do to you.

I consulted with the Gynecologist that was on call that day and had blood drawn. She took a detailed history (although there was not much to tell—no family history of breast or ovarian cancer, no weight gain, no bloating, etc). She told me that they would run my blood work and look for specific tumour markers that would confirm or deny exactly what they were suspecting. But she assured me and encouraged me to not go to a "dark place" yet, that it could potentially be something else—maybe just a benign mass. So, I walked out of the hospital that night clinging to what she said—and hanging onto a tiny thread of hope.

What I would realize in the coming months (and now years) is that I would need not just a tiny thread of hope but as much hope, strength, perseverance, persistence, and positivity as I could muster up... and then some. My blood work confirmed what the doctors had thought: I had metastatic ovarian cancer. I refused then or even now to capitalize those words, as I refuse to give them power or control over me. I learned first-hand that cancer does not discriminate against age, education, race, religion, or all be damned by how healthy you have lived your life. It can happen to any one of us at any time. It's hard to wrap your head around that, I know. It was one of the hardest things to accept for everyone (including me) when I was first diagnosed. When I was forced to tell my own patients that I had to take time off to undergo surgery and subsequently an intensive regimen of chemotherapy, many of them sat down, with tears streaming down their face, and said "How? You are the healthiest person we know."

I knew the upcoming battle was going to be hard, but I would tackle it the way that I had tackled everything else in my life: with a hard work ethic and a drive for success. I had been blessed with those qualities from a young age. I came from hardworking parents who were amazing role models. They taught me that "hard work pays off" and "nice matters." What I didn't know is how long this battle would be and how many times it would test me. I was ignorant of cancer and what cancer patients went through prior to my diagnosis. Sure, I knew of people who had also been diagnosed, but from an outsider looking in, I assumed it was straightforward: diagnosis, treatment, gone forever. I could do that. This, however, is not often the case, and has indeed not been my experience. I knew very little about ovarian cancer prior to my diagnosis. In reality, it was an organ to which I had rarely given much thought. I was never plagued by my monthly cycle with moodiness or cramps, nor had I made a conscious decision to try for kids yet.

So, they were tiny little organs that I had no connection with... until now. I only once read about ovarian cancer following my diagnosis. It was too difficult to read—grim, highest mortality rate, difficult to treat, poor prognosis. Honestly, who wants to read about that? And so I decided at that moment that I would not read any more about it on "Dr. Google." None of these articles knew ME, and I knew I was a unique and individual person—not a mere statistic—and I would not be defined in any other way.

In the early days after surgery, I never asked what stage I was categorized in, and to this day I have never asked a doctor about my prognosis or life expectancy. I don't find this information particularly helpful and cringe when someone else tells me that their doctor offered them this kind of information.

Really? Do they really know? Yes, they are doctors, but they are also only human.

Three weeks after I was diagnosed, I underwent extensive debulking surgery, which meant removing the tumour, any organs affected by it, and any trace of cancer that might be visible to the human eye. They moved quickly, as the cancer was "localized" and had not spread to distant sites. I was blessed with one of the province's best surgeons, and after 5 hours in the operating room I was tumour-free, but also had one less uterus, 2 less ovaries, was devoid of a greater omentum, and missing 5.5 inches of my large intestine. I was also the proud new owner (OK...maybe proud isn't the correct word) of an intraperitoneal port (IP) inserted just under my rib cage to be used in the next steps of my treatment plan. Just three weeks after surgery I started on what would ultimately be 18 straight weeks of chemotherapy: alternating one week in my veins and one week in my IP port. It was an aggressive attack. They told me this was my insurance policy—to attack and destroy any teeny, tiny cells that might still be floating around.

I believe that the first six months following any difficult life event is the hardest time to navigate—whether it be divorce, the death of a loved one, cancer, or even the joyous birth of a new baby. Ask anyone who has lived through any of these events and I think they would agree. You spend the first few days (sometimes weeks) in shock, and then as time slowly passes you start to learn to live with your "new normal." My experience was no different. When the initial shock of my diagnosis subsided, the fear slowly started to creep in and sometimes became overwhelming. I was suddenly faced with my own mortality, which is not something that any young, healthy person expects to face. As the fear eased ever so slightly, the feelings of loss hit like an ocean wave on Big Beach in Maui (if you know, you know!). I mourned the loss of my previous life...

my life before cancer.

For six months I did not go to work or teach a single fitness class. I missed the daily interactions with my coworkers, my patients, and all of the participants in my fitness classes; this was my life force and what fueled me every single day. My once-athletic body lost much of its muscle mass, and for the first time in my life I felt weak and vulnerable. My mind, which had always been my ally, now seemed to be my enemy. I felt like a foreigner in my own body and mind. It's hard to precisely recall how long I felt like this (maybe a few weeks? a month or two?) before I started to see more clearly. I started focusing my energy on what I could control, which I realized was, in fact, my body and mind. I flooded my body with healthy foods, juices, and rituals that made me feel alive (infrared sauna sessions, walks in nature, visits with friends, epsom salt baths, acupuncture appointments, vitamin IVs, and even the odd retail therapy excursion to the mall). I immersed my mind in books written by others who had walked a similar path or by researchers that offered hope to people going through cancer like me. I even focused my energy on fundraising and raising money for an organization that focuses specifically on ovarian cancer research and offering help to other women standing in my exact shoes. I knew that these things may not be the cure to my plight, but I also knew without a doubt that they helped me during the difficult moments. They reminded me that I was still alive, that I could still find joy in every day, and that despite all the losses I had experienced over the last six months, the one thing that cancer could not steal from me was hope—and my will to live.

What I already knew in my life BC (before cancer) was confirmed as I went through this journey and in the daily reminders from the people around me. I was reminded that what you put out into the universe, or to your community/your tribe, will come back to you tenfold in the times that you need it most.

Their messages were clear and they came in every possible form—emails, text messages, airplane rides and visits, snail mail cards, gift baskets, Amazon Prime deliveries, flowers, fundraisers, etc. Each time, the message to me was the same: "We've got your back; we'll hold you up when you feel weak; we are HERE for you." It was this massive outpouring of love that kept me going and reaffirmed to me that HOPE is more powerful than fear, that TOGETHER is better than alone, and that LOVE can heal all.

It sounds nice, right? That love can heal all. And it can, kinda sorta. It heals your heart, your mind, and yes, for some people, even their body. I remained cancer-free or NED (no evidence of disease) for just shy of three years before facing a recurrence. I knew that this was a possibility, but every part of my being had hoped and prayed that my journey was behind me. My life had resembled some sort of normalcy for those years but there were distinct differences now. I was back to work but with a more balanced approach to work and life, and I had traded in my high intensity fitness regime for the odd yoga class and many nature walks with my adorable goldendoodle. (Yes, he was my healing gift to myself when I finished my first round of treatment! Aside: if you are reading this and thinking that you need a dog in your life—YOU DO! The love is undescribable).

This recurrence put me back in the ring with another surgery and a few more rounds of chemo. But it also taught me lessons in positivity—that even on our darkest days, we need to look for the light. It taught me lessons in perseverance—that even when it may seem like you are out of options and can't keep going, you always have options. Finally, it taught me lessons in persistence—that you must always advocate for your own health (don't take no for an answer) and seek out and create the best medical team for yourself (get 2nd and even 3rd opinions). Essentially, create a medical team that wants you to beat this just as much as you do. I did this by connecting with others who inspired me and were on similar journeys, as well as researching what other treatments in Canada and overseas were out there that could potentially be life-saving for me.

As I write this chapter, I am still battling this disease every day... and I am "handling my hard stuff like a boss." The two most common questions I am asked, usually by friends or a patient, are: what has cancer taught me and how do I stay so positive and happy in the face of such adversity? First and foremost, it taught me that, hands-down, THE most important thing in this life—your life—is to take care of yourself, both mentally and physically. We have all heard the saying "you can't pour from an empty cup" and this couldn't be more true. We must prioritize our own health and take care of ourselves first before we focus on others. This was a difficult lesson for me initially, as I truly believe that I was born a healer with a generosity of giving. Helping someone else by easing their physical suffering or boosting their mental wellness gave me great pride and satisfaction in my own life and work, but in hindsight I saw that it was at the expense of my own health.

What does prioritizing your own health look like? It is more than just a spa day or a trip to the mall for some retail therapy (although both are nice!). It means to fuel your body with healthy food (salads, smoothies, green juices, plant-based diet), choosing a balanced approach to exercise (nourish, not punish, workout days vs. rest days). It involves taking care of your body on the inside as much as you do the outside—drinking tons of water, avoiding toxins (what you put on your body goes in your body), detoxing (infrared sauna sessions, warm epsom salt baths, and cold showers or plunges) all with the same goal of minimizing inflammation in our bodies. I adopted all of these new lifestyle habits (easy to embrace when you are faced with life or death) and I can honestly say that I look and feel better and healthier than I did before my diagnosis. I have more energy, a fresh glow to my skin, and overall less inflammation in my body.

Prioritizing your health doesn't just mean your physical health; it is taking care of your mental fitness as well. I did this by reading inspiring books, watching inspirational videos, and using one of the many meditation apps on the market, and, perhaps more important than all of these, I surrounded myself with the best support crew a girl could ask for. I can tell you from first-hand experience that there are so many "helpers" in this world and people genuinely want to help others. I have been blessed by my family and friends who have leveled up and carried me forward on this journey. Facing any hard life event ALONE will undoubtedly make the event that much more difficult. If you are facing hardship while reading this, look for the helpers in your life, lean on your friends and family when things get tough, or reach out to a support group of people who are going through the same life event as you. As the saying goes, you will find strength in numbers. I was blown away by the massive outpouring of love that I have received from everyone in my life throughout this journey—even those I had lost contact with who reached out when they heard of my struggle.

As the receiver of such love and support, I am reminded that there is so much good in this world, AND that I can also reach out and support others when they are going through hard times. The reality is that we will ALL face adversity in our lifetime, and if we can lessen the pain others feel, we should do whatever it takes to do that.

As I mentioned above, the second most common question that I have been asked is how I remain so positive and happy every single day. My answer is always the same: there is always something to be grateful for. A life altering journey like this always puts what is important into laser focus. You learn what and who is important to you. You stop sweating the small stuff and focus on what is REALLY important in your life. I find joy in things that I didn't even notice before, like the sun shining between the trees in an old growth forest, or how precious time is spent with a friend just having a coffee or a stroll. Truth be told, I wish we could learn these important things without facing a major life crisis, but unfortunately most of us need a wake up call to really appreciate what is important and what we have. To maintain my positivity and happiness I also just try and handle things one day at a time. It may sound cliché, but that's really all any of us can do. We take life one day at a time and try not to predict our future, as none of us really knows what the outcome of our life will be. We can only control so much and we have to find peace and comfort that we have done everything possible that is within our control, and then we leave the rest up to fate.

As a healthcare professional, woman, and now cancer warrior, I feel compelled—actually, obligated—to finish this chapter by reiterating the importance of listening to your body, going with your gut, and following your intuition. Do not ignore or dismiss any abnormal symptoms that you may be experiencing. Make an appointment with your doctor and get it checked out. As scary as it can be, remember that knowledge is power, and in conditions like cancer, most types, if caught early, are curable. In regards to ovarian cancer, there are no reliable tests that can be done preventatively (No...that test we all lovvvve *does not detect ovarian cancer)*, and the symptoms are vague and often mimic other things. This is why it is even more important than ever to listen to what your body is telling you. If you have bloating, pelvic or abdominal (belly) pain, trouble eating or feeling full quickly, or urinary symptoms such as urgency (always feeling like you have to go) or frequency (having to go often) and any of these symptoms last more than 3 weeks, I plead with you to go and see a medical professional. If my story can save just one person then everything I have gone through to date is worth it.

It would be a stretch to say that cancer is a gift or that I wouldn't change a thing about how my life has unfolded thus far. I don't believe anyone going through this would say that. But what I can say is that there are blessings in every battle and that the last chapter of my life has not been written, so I will continue to live each day with grace and gratitude. My hope is that you will do the same.

Chapter 7
JENNA PETERS

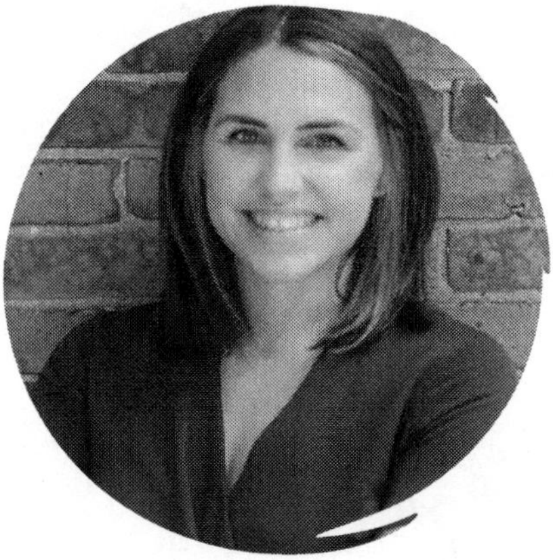

Photographer: Monika Parr / Monika Parr Photography

Instagram @jpeters01
j.miles3@hotmail.com

The feeling was surreal. Unimaginable. Like a bad accident you can't look away from. It felt like a literal bomb had gone off and I was in the middle of a war. Time stood still, my vision tunelled, and everything around me went dark. The entire memory is dark. Panic and fear paralyzed my limbs. I couldn't move; I couldn't think; I couldn't act. All that I could do was stare at his lifeless body.

This felt like hours of paralyzation when in reality it was seven minutes. Seven minutes! When I looked back at the call info, I could hardly believe it. There's no way. There must be a mistake. It felt like I was down in that basement for hours, just panicking and pacing and swearing. PTSD is a powerful thing.

It felt as though my brain had left my body. I could see myself panicking. I could hear all of my thoughts as if I were saying them out loud, but the room was silent. There was a haze of heaviness that fell over everyone.

My body was acting almost robotic. Check pulse, start CPR, get the monitor, call for backup, get the hell out of there. My body was just moving without cue and I was just watching, out of body.

Have you ever heard those stories about near-death experiences and when the person tells the story, they describe someone who saved them—but they weren't actually there? For a few days after the call I questioned this. During what felt like a trance, a man walked down the stairs. He heard the call over his radio and voluntarily chose to bring this trauma into his life. Had he not, I don't know where I would be. It's worth mentioning that he was wearing a white tactical shirt. It was like a bright beam of light walked down those stairs. You can see the angel-like vibes I questioned. He had a sense of calmness to him. It felt as though he could hear everything I was thinking. He carried me through the rest of that day... those seven minutes in the basement, the drive to the hospital, the moments following. I will never forget this man.

The moments following are a blur. I felt desperate for help. I was gripping onto everything and everyone I could until I could make it home to my husband and kids. It was like a scene out of a movie. I walked out of those hospital doors, sat down out of sight, and just let it all out.

Mat leave was a blur. With two kids 17 months apart life was a damn blur. I was looking forward to heading back to work as a medic and feeling a different sense of purpose apart from motherhood—and if I'm being completely honest, having a break from the chaos at home. I started back at the end of May 2019, on my son's birthday. I was feeling anxious and all types of things going back to paramedics after a year of momming.

Going back to shift work as a mom of two was an adjustment on it's own. I was missing morning snuggles, bedtime stories, and all of the chaos in between. I wouldn't see the kids for four or five days at a time. The guilt was heavy on my heart.

After my second child, I was feeling all types of things that I didn't quite understand at the time. I had no connection to my son and I felt so much guilt for it. I chalked it up to growing up with a sister and my daughter never having those same memories. Little did I know, I was suffering from postpartum depression—the resentment, the lack of connection, the guilt, all of it.

I resented my little boy for taking time away from my daughter, who was only 17 months at the time and needed all of me. I felt guilty for feeling guilty, and it was this vicious cycle. I would talk up the love for my son in hopes that people didn't see through me...

...until my life took a completely different direction that I naively never saw coming.

My feet were still miles off the ground. All I kept telling myself was, "just get home, just get home and you'll be okay." The sun was hot. I had already changed into my regular clothes and left all my belongings in my locker. Little did I know that was the last time that I would step foot in that place.

That morning I showed up to work like any other shift, with two coffees in hand: one for the hour drive, the other for when I got there. I put my lunch away and began my regular morning routine. I unpacked my work gear, checked the truck, and booked on for the day.

Not more than an hour later, the tones went off. This was the moment that my life went spiraling down another path that I had for some reason never anticipated.

I know what you're thinking: "You're a paramedic, how did you not expect to see such awful things?" Well, let me tell you, nothing can prepare you for what your specific trauma is. To some, it's the teenager who took the corner too fast, to others it's domestic abuse, and to me it was a little boy who never woke up.

I remember my literal call for help walking out of the hospital that day, knowing that I wasn't okay. I was feeling everything crumbling inside of me. I was grateful to have two incredible supervisors know exactly what I needed before I even knew what was going on. They were there to guide me through the moments I felt like I couldn't stand. They sat with me for hours until my feet came back to the ground and I could drive myself home. Home to my son.

It's hard to know what is going to tip your bucket over. It can be 14,250 little things and one minor little drop that sets you off, or it can be one giant tsunami that fills it up all at once. I was the latter.

I was not okay. I knew I was not okay. The second I got home I remember running to the backyard and desperately needing my son. It felt like I had longed for this moment in so many ways, on so many levels—needing to hold him, touch him, look at him, cry with him. He had no idea of the storm inside of me. We all hadn't a clue what we were in for.

This is my story about momming through PTSD.

The days after that call are a blur. I could still feel the panic and fear that I felt in those moments of the call. I was afraid to be alone. I couldn't be alone. I laid on the couch and cried. I needed to talk, to cry, to scream. There would be lapses in time when my mind would wander to what was on the T.V. or what the kids were fighting over, and within seconds it would bounce back to my reality—to what I couldn't unsee but wished so badly that I could. Everything seemed like a haze—almost like an eclipse—where it's light out but there is this creepy, shadowy, cathartic haze over your life. I needed to talk; I needed to cry; I needed to scream.

My first psych appointment was the day after the call. I was anxious and afraid. I was afraid to drive there myself, to talk about what still felt like a dream, and to attempt to drive home. After six months of therapy, I felt as though I hadn't even made a dent in my progress. I felt completely unsupported and misunderstood. There was a brief moment of panic that ensued again. Where do I go now? How do I start all over? Can I even mentally handle starting over?

I made the switch to a new therapist who ultimately is the reason that I am where I am now. She explained to me what I was feeling: the irritability, the constant fear, the pain. I wasn't "crazy." I wasn't a "bad mom." I wasn't selfish. I was grieving... grieving the loss of someone I never knew. Someone my family never knew. And it took almost a year for me to understand that that was okay.

I remember laying in bed in October, two months after that day. There was a weird thunder storm, awkwardly late in the season. The thunder boomed, and I remember feeling panic strike. My body seized up and I could feel the pulses in my arms, which made them feel tingly and numb. My heart felt like it might beat right out of my chest. I cried... I cried so hard. I had no idea what was going on. I woke up my husband in a panic, in fear. It was a fear so surreal that it brought me back to that day so quickly... to the fear that I had felt in those moments.

There were several things in the coming months that brought me back to that day. My son had a little tumble around the pool that summer. His nose was bleeding. Pretty minor first aid was required. I've seen it a million times. I knew that he just needed a snuggle. As soon as he started walking towards me crying with blood dripping from his nose, I froze. I felt so nauseated and lightheaded. I screamed for my husband to come down so that I could escape from the situation. I ran inside to the bathroom to try to breathe through the nausea. My head started pounding. Seriously? I couldn't handle snuggling away my baby's bumps anymore? What was happening?

Another time an Amber Alert had gone off while we were relaxing in bed. My arms went numb, my heart was pounding, and I felt so much fear surge through my body.

What was this? I hadn't gone to war. I wasn't ducking at the sound of gunfire. I felt ridiculous. I felt afraid. I felt alone. I felt like a completely different person. I avoided social media so that I didn't scroll across any child-related news stories. I avoided the news. I avoided messages. I felt so far from myself that I lost sight of myself.

Enough time had passed that I started to question if I would ever be my happy, bubbly self again. I questioned whether therapy was even working. I was off work, with no direction or end game. I had no idea where I was going or what I was doing. I was lost—trying to be a good mom, a good wife, a good friend. I was so irritable with everyone and everything—swearing at inanimate objects, slamming cupboards, kicking toys. I felt like the memory of that day was less frequent. The dreams had calmed down. I thought that meant that I had made progress. Little did I know, my threshold was still so high. I had no idea that just because the memories were fewer, it didn't mean they had been processed or gone anywhere. They were just below the surface, holding me back from… well, me.

My kids needed me; my husband needed me; and simply put, I wasn't home. Luckily my husband spent 15 years as a paramedic. He knew exactly what I needed. He was so patient. I remember the first night after I got home and he had put the kids to bed, just laying there on the couch staring, crying, trying to forget. I remember him misunderstanding what I said and thinking I wanted to be alone. He started walking upstairs to go to bed, and I will never forget the fear that came over me. It was a fear like I was smack dab in the middle of a horror flick and the wind was about to blow open a window and an axe murderer was going to pop out from the shadows. That kind of fear. I snapped. "Where are you going??!!" He stopped mid-stair and said, "I thought you wanted to be alone." I just started crying. "I said I don't want to be alone!" I pleaded hysterically like my life was in danger. He laid there with me for hours. When he would hear me cry, he would comfort me. When I started to stare off, he would talk to me. He was everything I needed in that moment and all the moments we would go through together after that first night. He made up for everything I lacked in the weeks following.

I couldn't eat without feeling guilt. I couldn't sleep without feeling guilt. I couldn't smile without feeling guilt. It was a guilt so heavy it made me nauseous. I felt guilt for being alive when he wasn't. I would spend the nights with my son in his toddler bed just laying there watching him. Noting every little wrinkle in his face, watching his chest rise and fall, holding his hands until I fell asleep with him in his little bed. I had never felt so drained in my entire life—not after two natural births, not after shift work and a cranky baby, not from anything. My head was spinning endlessly.

It's a hard feeling to understand. A piece of me wants to completely forget that day—to have some type of stroke that only affects that specific memory. The other piece of me knows that if I rewrote that day, I wouldn't be where I am right now: free, healthy, and with direction.

After another few months with my new therapist, working through it all step-by-step and trying to make sense of what I was going through, I began a new type of therapy.

Exposure therapy scared the hell out of me, especially almost a year later. I had gotten good at pushing it down—summing up into a few sentences why I was off work and carrying on with my day. I had to; I was a mom. My kids needed dinner and baths and story time. They needed me. Looking back, I was a shell of a human at that point; hating bath time because it was chaotic, dreading dinner and bedtime because I would just be up all night anyway.

When I met my occupational therapist, I was terrified of having to go into detail about that day all over again. After our first appointment, she thanked me. She thanked me for having the courage to go down this road and for sharing that day with her in so much detail. No one had verbally appreciated my pain before. I knew this was the beginning of a new path.

At first we worked on very basic things... or so I thought. We worked on sleep patterns, healthy habits—all of the things that I had lost, whether from unpredictable shift work life, or from that day. The cause didn't matter; these basic things were the foundation—and mine had crumbled. She held me accountable and I didn't want to disappoint her.

After a few weeks, we got into the heavier side of exposure therapy. We sat down and wrote out a list of all of the things that I had been avoiding in the last year, on a scale from 1-10... 10 being "I would rather spend the night in a haunted mansion than face said exposure." We listed them one by one. My anxiety and fear rose the higher we climbed up the list. I remember sitting there realizing the things I'd avoided for the last year: my favourite podcast I used to listen to on the way to work, my pool shed where my uniforms hid in black garbage bags poking through from little holes in the bags, a highway. It started "small": sitting and listening to the podcast with my therapist. Feeling the feels in that moment, sitting with them, being uncomfortable. We slowly moved up the list. As each week went on, I knew we were one exposure closer to my number 10: having to drive back to where it all happened.

The first time we drove there, I had no idea if I even remembered the route. I just got in my car and drove. Once we got there, I had no idea where I was going to stop. The specific spot? Somewhere in sight of it? Somewhere else all together? I just shut my brain off and drove. I stopped within sight, pulled over, and turned my car off. We got out and just walked. We walked around the block and chatted like friends. When we got back to the car I almost forgot where I was. I was calm, I was aware, and I was okay... enough. We spent many more visits there, talking, writing, and feeling safe in a place I once felt fear.

You don't get into Paramedics thinking about the day you're going to leave. You put everything you have into becoming one. School, ride outs, shift work, job processes, lift tests, practicals. You don't plan a backup because you don't have any room for doubt. Yet here I am, knowing I am never going back to my career as a paramedic, with no backup plan, two kids, and a husband figuring out his own path. We were not in a financial position for me to go back to school, and the two kids sort of put a strain on college at 30. I had to find happiness outside of a career. It took months to wrap my head around a mundane career, a 9-to-5 office job, two days off a week with my kids, rush hour, and, I'm assuming, CHFI playing in the background. But you know what I realized? It was a hell of a lot better than where I was. It was a hell of a lot brighter than any path I had been on before. And who knows, maybe I'd finally win one of those midday radio contests.

There was no clear moment when I realized I was on the other side—no double rainbow arches, no yellow brick road. Life just started to feel a little more normal. The thoughts were less frequent and when they did pop in, they were more comforting than intrusive. The memories were beautiful. They became lighter.

I used to describe the memory in colour. I sometimes see things like that—a vibe, if you will. I used to tell my therapist that the memory was cigarette-stained yellow. Any time thoughts or visions made their way past my attempt to dodge them, they were cigarette-stained yellow. It felt icky, and I felt icky—like a horror movie you're watching through your fingers. (Or at least that's how I watch them, with the blur of my fingers in my face.)

My kids may never know why we have cupcakes on random days throughout the year or why mommy isn't herself sometimes when memories intrude, but they will grow up with the best me because of this day. They will grow up with a mom who wasn't afraid to veer off her path. A mom who persevered and powered through. A mom who wasn't afraid to break down and cry with her kids, but knew when to stand up and make dinner.

A mom who wasn't afraid to ask for help.

It's been a struggle writing this. I'm currently on the outs of therapy and I've associated that with the outs of this whole experience. But that day has changed my life forever, for the better. Cliché, right? But if the "Men in Black" offered me an electro bio-mechanical neural transmitting zero synapses repositioner, I'd turn that shit down. It's not a matter of overcoming the trauma, but learning how to carry it a little better. Much like carrying all of the groceries and your flailing toddlers into the house at the same time, you just get better at it. It's learning how to take that experience and dig out all of the opportunities that it's hiding.

I needed help. I needed it on so many different levels. I needed help taking care of my kids, and keeping up with all of the things that life still carries on with when you're on the couch grieving. My husband, my family, and my friends kept me treading above water. It definitely was not lifeguard training, hands up, shoulders above water treading—but I was afloat enough. Afloat enough to see everyone advocating for me when I didn't have it in me, afloat enough to see my husband help carry the weight of this pain, and afloat enough to make it through.

Don't get me wrong, there are still days. Days that the memory becomes too much and I literally shake my head to try and throw it off as if it's going to just fly out of my ears. Days I'm irritable because my threshold is just too high and my bucket spills over before I've even had my coffee. But I'm mindful of it. I acknowledge the thought and *abracadabra* it away. Because I have the power to do that. I have the power to control my thoughts and how I perceive them.

I'm grateful that I came out on the other side. I am forever grateful for what this experience has brought my son and I. Whether it was gratitude for his life, or acknowledging my postpartum struggle and overcoming it, I don't know. But it changed something between us that is hard to put into words. We have a connection that beams through my heart, one we didn't have before. I'm grateful for all of the doors that flew open once I accepted this new path. I'm grateful that I was aware enough to fully embrace them. The unknown is always going to be a little unsettling, but isn't it possible that it's a hell of a lot better than where you were?

So I leave you with this: leave your brain some room for the possibility that it IS going to work out. You don't have to believe everything happens for a reason or believe in fate, but just base it off your life stats. Base it off how you got to where you are now. I know the self-belief gets a little lost, but there are always tidbits of hope trying to poke through, even if just for a second.

Take those moments and hold on tight. Let them lead you; they know what the f*ck they're doing. Don't be afraid to recruit a village to mosh pit you through it, because looking back, I don't know what I would have done without my village. I think in desperation you'd find it anywhere... survival mode for your family, for your kids. But I credit a lot of where I am now to it. The therapists that all nudged me in the right direction, the occupational therapist with tough love who became almost a friend and forced me to face the uncomfortable, and the family that allowed me to grieve in my own way regardless of what that looked like.

I'm okay... enough. That day will always leave a sour taste, but the route it paved was worth all of the pain. It may feel like you're driving down Eglinton Ave. E, but I promise that there will be a day when you're driving top down on Rodeo Drive with paparazzi snapping photos of this beautiful new you. When you're ready to embrace the doors, they'll open. When you're ready to smile again, you will. When you're ready to accept the new you, the stronger you, the better you, you will. Plus, Sour Patch Kids are pretty sweet once you power through the sour.

Chapter 8

ML

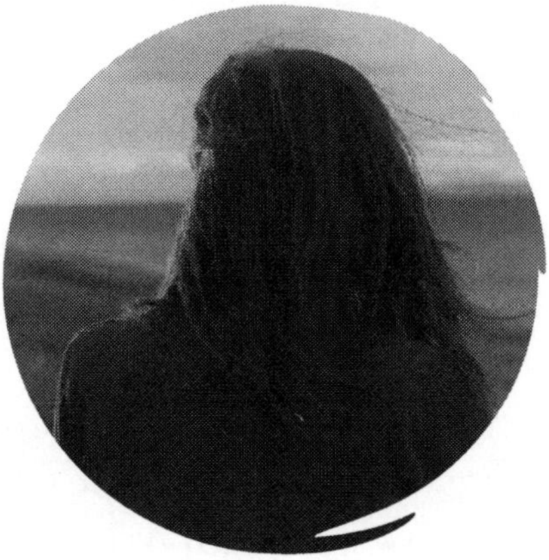

It was June 2011. I had just completed four years of my undergraduate degree in Forensic Science followed by one year of Teacher's College. I was in the driveway at my parents' house, about to get into the car to start the first day of my new job. I remember quickly reminiscing on the past five years—the countless hours in the library, the labs, essays, courses, practicums, struggles, triumphs, and tribulations that had brought me to that moment in time. I distinctly recall the thought in my head that this must be happening for a reason, as contrary to seemingly everyone else's expectations, I had not yet acquired a career in my field. I acknowledged that I was not where I imagined I would be, but I shrugged my shoulders and drove to a wing restaurant to start my first shift as a waitress.

Work was tough; my manager was one of the angriest people

I have ever encountered. I was apprehensive, but still showed up every day to spend 12 hours on my feet, often serving alone without a break or time to eat. I knew this position would be temporary, and I just wanted to quickly pay off my student debt from Teacher's College. I was usually granted one or two days off per week. However, the manager would usually send me a message desperately asking me to come in to work on my days off. I would rarely say no, despite the energy in that environment being dismal.

In November 2011, a group of construction workers came into the restaurant. I noticed that one guy seemed to be staring at me. When he came up to the register to pay his bill, he handed me a wet nap packet with his name and number on it and said, "If you'd like to go out some time, call me." We started talking, and by January 2012, he was my boyfriend.

My boyfriend—Jay—was assisting with the construction of the hospital down the street from where I was working. He was thoughtful, funny, and caring. We spoke often and enjoyed each other's company. He lived an hour out of town, so we tried to see each other every possible moment we could. I thought that finding each other was the reason that I was supposed to work at the restaurant; He was the silver lining in a dark cloud.

Jay was a hard worker. He would often express his exhaustion after working 16-hour days and had little time off to recover. I told him that if he didn't take it easy, he would get hurt. In February 2012, that's exactly what happened. He was loading up his truck at work and hundreds of pounds of scaffolding material fell onto him. He braced the impact with his hand (trying to push the materials off of him) and his knee. For days he complained about being in pain, but stubbornly refused to go to the doctor. After about a week, I finally convinced him to go to the hospital. He walked out with a cast on his left wrist. He was living in an apartment at the time, and I stayed with him more to help him out. This eventually led to me moving out of my parents' house and living with him full time early on in our relationship.

The injury significantly impacted Jay's attitude. He was sad, moody, and constantly expressing how much pain he was in. I did my best to console him and tried to make him comfortable, but my efforts were inconsequential when seemingly nothing helped, and he was unwilling to take his medication as prescribed. He wouldn't sleep at night and would toss and turn. After a couple of months, Jay's cast was removed and he could not move his hand. I knew something was terribly wrong. The slightest touch of the skin over his wrist would make him fall to his knees in tears. He explained his pain as feeling like electricity shooting through his wrist, and there was no doubt in my mind that it was excruciating.

Jay began seeing a specialist who eventually diagnosed him with Chronic Regional Pain Syndrome. We were advised that it was as a result of his cast being on for too long. Additionally, there was a tear between the two carpals in his wrist. Despite desperately needing it, Jay was not a candidate for surgery due to his immense pain and having zero range of motion in his hand.

Jay had countless appointments with various medical professionals, but little progress was made as they were unable to touch his wrist. Days of pain turned into months. I spent every single day living with him, feeling helpless while watching him suffer in chronic pain. I knew exactly what movements would hurt him and truly felt like I could feel the pain myself sometimes. I felt so isolated during this time, like I was trapped in a nightmare. I was working in a less than ideal environment and going home to someone in agony. Since Jay was injured so early into our relationship, we never really had the opportunity to connect or have fun in a social environment. Friends and family would express sympathy, but did not fully appreciate the severity of the situation. This relationship was not what I pictured it would be when I first met him, but I did not have the heart to leave. I loved him, was the only person who could take care of him, and we had been through so much together in a short period of time. I held onto a glimmer of hope that once he recovered, we could give it a real chance.

Jay was unable to attend work and was receiving minimal income through insurance. Every phone call with the insurance company seemed like a battle and would exacerbate his frustration and pain. It was insulting and demeaning when some people suggested he was faking his injury. We eventually discovered Jay was being observed and followed by a Private Investigator. I continued to work at the restaurant, and eventually left that position for another similar job. We managed to make ends meet, and I covered the bulk of the expenses.

After months of little to no progress, the Doctor ordered Jay to attend weekly nerve block injections. This entailed Jay receiving a large needle inserted in the front of his neck which extended to the back of his spine, and injecting medication around a bundle of nerves to temporarily relieve the pain. The first two days after Jay had this procedure were the only moments that I witnessed him experience some form of relief and the physiotherapist was able to touch and move his wrist. I remember being shocked the first time I saw someone touch his wrist without him screaming. The pain had been persistent for so long, it was inconceivable to me that it would ever subside.

After nine or ten rounds of the nerve block and countless appointments to physio, he was finally able to move his hand enough that he was eligible for surgery. This was three years after his initial injury.

After surgery, Jay continued rehabilitation and was gradually able to move his wrist to make almost a full recovery; it was truly a miracle. Our lives slowly started improving, and there was finally hope for good times ahead. In honour of Jay's recovery, we took a celebratory cruise to the Caribbean. Jay eventually enrolled in a course to be a Private Investigator and acquired a career in the field shortly after. I went back to school for Emergency Telecommunications and obtained a position as a 911 dispatcher. Initially I was commuting one hour to work, and we eventually moved closer so I was only 30 minutes away. We adopted two dogs, had a lot of laughs, and started going on fun adventures that we couldn't do when he was injured.

Jay's work was steady throughout the spring and fall, but dwindled in the winter. Jay and I did not realize this would be the case. It was during this time that I started picking up more of the bills—not thinking anything of it—because Jay reassured me the work lull would be temporary.

The following year the same thing happened, except this time Jay said he would pick up a seasonal job to supplement his income. He never followed through. I didn't realize the extent of Jay's financial struggles at the time, as they were masked by him being off work due to his injury. It was a red flag that I didn't see.

This unsteady work cycle went on for about four years until he got into an argument with his supervisor. It's still not super clear to me whether he quit or resigned, but regardless, the burden of paying the bills fell solely on me again. Jay made a lot of promises about acquiring work and often spoke about the businesses that he wanted to start. I believed he would accomplish his career goals because the injury was no longer a burden to his progress. He spoke about his plans confidently and he had so much potential to be great. Unfortunately, he never followed through with any of his ideas.

Jay started asking me to borrow money. In the beginning he would always pay me back, but eventually he wasn't able to because he was unable to maintain steady employment. It got to the point where I could not rely on him. I thought about leaving him many times, but quickly realized it was not as easy as it sounds on paper when you are living with someone. All I could envision was having to pay rent and all of the bills where we were living, in addition to trying to come up with first and last month's rent on a new place where I would live alone. I thought I had nowhere to go and kept myself trapped thinking the grass would not be greener on the other side.

By January 2019, Jay had accumulated significant debt and because we were together, I looked at his debt as being my own. I encouraged him to apply for jobs, but he always had some excuse about why he wasn't working. He believed he was overqualified for many positions and refused to work for less money than he felt like he was worth. Ultimately, his poor work ethic and lack of discipline meant more financial instability.

I started picking up more shifts to the point that I became addicted to working overtime. Every day I would obsess over checking what extra shifts were available and craved the seconds of relief I felt when I successfully signed up for them, knowing at least one more bill would be taken care of. I was not able to relax and lived in a state of mental and physical exhaustion. I was willing to do whatever it took—sacrificing my well-being and my ability to be present with friends and family during the minimal time I had available to spend with them.

I was so physically drained that some days I could only muster up the energy to move to go to work. Working an unpredictable combination of day and night shifts made me feel like a zombie. I was so distracted and overwhelmed by our financial situation, I did not realize the toll this had taken on my mental health. I had become depressed, began questioning life, and though I never had a plan to kill myself, I began to see death as my only way out. I never imagined something like this would happen to me, and I wasn't sure how to get out of this dark place. I expressed this to Jay many times, but it wasn't enough for him to make the necessary changes to help balance our relationship. I would be working away while he was home playing video games or out fishing with friends. I flashed back to that moment in 2011 before going to work in the restaurant, and realized how far I had come and how much I had been through. I had worked hard and knew this relationship was never what I had imagined for myself and my future. Something had to change.

I remember one day in September 2020 I was driving to work for a night shift. I was exhausted and started bawling as I was driving; I think it was a combination of the sun making my eyes water combined with my emotions of tiredness and resentment. I had reached my breaking point. I remember saying out loud, "God, if I'm not supposed to be in this relationship, please, please take me out of it."

A few days later my brother and sister-in-law invited my mom and I over for a visit. We were drinking tea in their sunroom after dinner. Somehow, the topic came up about Jay. My family expressed their concerns about his inability to maintain work and a steady income, and could see the obvious toll it was taking on me. I brushed them off, thinking I was concerned too, but wasn't sure what they expected me to do when I had nowhere to go. My sister-in-law said I was welcome to stay with them. That was a pivotal moment in my life. I realized that due to my embarrassment about the situation and desire to protect him, it had never occurred to me to tell anyone about my struggles, or to ask for help to get out of the relationship. I did not expect her offer to mean that I would be leaving him a few days later, but my family and I came up with a plan for me to get out. It was surreal.

My prayer was answered on September 25, 2020. This was the hardest day of my life. The night before Jay had asked me if I loved him and I said that I did. I didn't sleep well and remembered waking up feeling sick to my stomach, wondering how I was going to follow through with leaving him. He called me downstairs to eat breakfast that he had made for me. I couldn't act normal and started crying. When he asked me what was wrong, I finally said the words: "I am leaving." He pleaded and begged for one more chance. I had given him one more chance every day for eight-and-a-half years.

I told him that I couldn't stay and that doing so was only enabling him to not grow or make progress in his own life. My brother and sister-in-law arrived shortly after and helped me pack my stuff—primarily clothes. Over time I continued to gather more of my belongings. Leaving was harder than I ever imagined and it soon occurred to me that all the work it took was what I was avoiding for so long. I paid for everything—the rent, both of our bills, his debt, everything. To this day, he doesn't understand why I left, because though he was taking advantage of me, he wasn't intentionally using me for money or anything else.

I lived with my brother for four months. I am very grateful for the assistance and can honestly say I wouldn't be where I am without them. However, living there did come with its own challenges and adaptations. No one knew me like Jay did—and no one knew him like I did. People around me were supportive, but seemingly hated when I brought him up. They expected me to just move on and forget about him. Though I have no desire to get back together with him, I can't escape nearly a decade of memories with him. You don't necessarily realize how much of your identity is wrapped up in someone else until they are removed. Often the only person I would want to help me feel better about breaking up with him—was him.

In February 2021, I ended up moving out of my brother's house and into a new place on my own. In the beginning, it didn't feel as good as I thought it would. I was very depressed and sought counselling. It took me about a year to feel better. Jay got to stay in the house we were living in with many of the things I had worked hard to accumulate over the past eight-and-a-half years. I had already lost so much (physically, emotionally, and financially) being with him, but leaving him felt like I had lost even more.

What I gained, however, is much more important than anything materialistic ever will be: a new beginning and a second chance to get it right. I discovered that sometimes the grass is indeed greener on the other side. Looking back, I know I did everything in my power to make our relationship work—to the point that I didn't want to live anymore. It was still not enough to make him change or pull his weight. Never settle for less than what you deserve, and don't be afraid to ask for help. Thank you to every single person who supported me in this hard-won battle. You were the wind in my sails and I wouldn't be here without you.

Chapter 9
MICHELLE PFILE

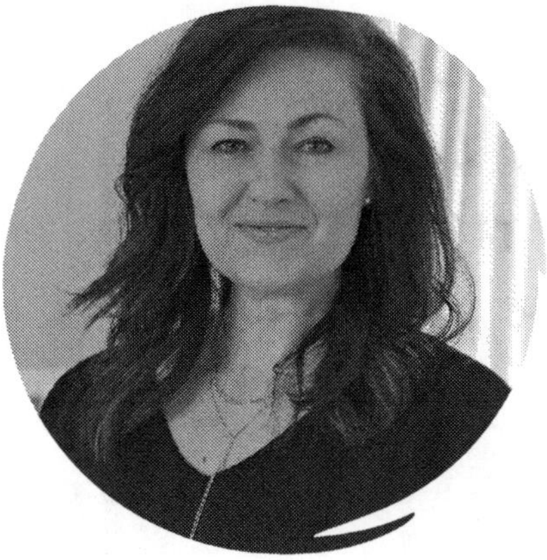

Photographer: Niki Patel

Instagram @itsmichellepfile
www.michellepfile.com

It was a normal morning. I'd just brushed my teeth, piled my hair on top of my head, and put on my workout gear. Suddenly I whipped around and caught my reflection in the mirror.

I made a hard lock with my eyes. Those eyes... it was like I was seeing them for the first time in months, and they looked so foreign to me, almost like they belonged to a stranger.

Those were tired eyes... glazed over and foggy. I stood there, locked in, paralyzed for longer than I'd looked at myself in a full year, and then they started.

The tears that encompassed six years of *hard* started to fall.

They fell for what seemed like hours, unleashing years of anger, sadness, frustration... tears of exhaustion. Completely devastated tears. I was so tired. Tired of being angry, sad, confused, and distant.

October 7, 2018—almost two years after the fact—was the day that I broke wide open.

I was really irritated. It was the week before Christmas for goodness sake. Why now? Why did it have to be right now? I had so much going on.

I was finishing up my 20+ year career as a hairstylist, and I was finally going to be able to devote all of my energy to my three-year-old online business. I had made the decision that my career as a hairstylist was over, and I was so excited!

On top of that, I was also a mom to a four-year-old, who naturally was excited for the season. We were building a house, and did I mention it was Christmas? WHY NOW???!

I was so pissed. This wasn't the first time that we'd done this song and dance... go to the hospital, assume this was the end, prepare ourselves, say our goodbyes over and over (AGAIN), and end up bringing my Dad home by some freak miracle... and he'd be good as new for another six months to a year.

But why now? Why at Christmas?!

NUMB. Disbelief.

I sat beside the bed in the critical care unit with my mom and brother—and I watched the clock, tick tock. It was 11:50 p.m. on Christmas Eve. I wasn't angry anymore. I was just shocked.

He was actually going to die; this was actually it. It felt like a joke. I even made a few. My head was spinning, but I wasn't saying anything that was locked deep inside my heart. I couldn't get those words out. We sat there for what seemed like hours, not saying anything to him or to each other. We just sat there and waited.

At 12:01 a.m. on December 25, 2016, my Dad passed away after battling Stage 4 Lung Cancer for over five years.

Wait—what? He's gone? I had so much that I needed to say. All I could think was *I didn't get my chance, it all happened so fast, and I truly don't think I ever thought you would be gone. You don't die; you always survive.*

My father had survived a radical surgery never done before in our country. He survived 100 days in ICU and literally came back completely normal after weeks of not being able to talk, walk, or breathe on his own. We never thought it was possible that he'd be close to normal, but he came back better than ever... and NOW out of the blue it felt like he DIED?

It's Christmas.

We didn't have a warning. This isn't how it's supposed to be. This isn't how I planned it. I didn't have a chance to say good-bye... *Dad, I have to tell you something, ask you something...* all I kept thinking was *PLEASE wait!*

PLEASE... come back...

For the next few days the only thought that rolled through my mind as I completed all of the expected duties of a fatherless daughter was *I can't believe I will never ever talk to my Dad again...*

Game Face ON!

You're the mature one, Michelle. Everyone is counting on you. You have people to see, people to comfort, haul out the waterproof mascara, write the speech that you know will knock everyone's socks off, and handle it!

Animal print pencil skirt, hair and makeup flawless...GO!

Big smile, open arms, comfort others... that's all you need to do for three days, and then this will be over...

Hundreds of people... HUNDREDS OF PEOPLE!

You've got this!

"Yes, I know—he was such a good man..."

"Oh, I know you will miss him so much..."

"He thought the world of you too..."

"How's your mom doing?

"She's doing ok."

"It's so good you are so close by, for her..."

"Yes, yes it is."

"How's your brother doing? He has such big shoes to fill, it must be so hard on him..."

"Yes, he sure does. I know he'll miss Dad, but he's doing a great job..."

Speak to the people Michelle. Give them what you do best—a little sarcasm, a few giggles, and close it out with a sappy quote.

You've got this!

The party—why is there a party? It makes no sense. But here we go! Be the entertainer, speak to the people, feed them, comfort them—it's almost over... You've got this.

Bed at last—NUMB.

My name is Michelle Pfile. I'm a wife, mom, and an online entrepreneur. I found my absolute passion for helping women just seven years ago! I love working with women who are frustrated with their current circumstances—whether with their health and wellness, mindset, or finances. I teach skills that help women walk through the things that are holding them back from seeing massive success when they can't seem to get unstuck.

Sharing my story through social media and my top-rated podcast has been one of the ways that I've been able to connect with and help women, and now I hope that I'll be able to help you as you read my story. Maybe you'll relate to my words, feelings, and thoughts that I share them.

One thing that I know for sure, is that we will all encounter grief in our lives and we'll all lose someone who has meant that absolute world to us. When it happens, it may feel like you can't go on. I hope in some small way this will help you become aware of what may come, and give you some tools for your toolbox to the road back to yourself.

In the event that you find yourself in a similar situation as myself—feeling like you're in the darkest season of your life—one which no one understands and you don't even understand, know that I do. Remember this chapter and come back to it for comfort.

December 25, 2017

And just like that, I'd done it! I'd survived a FULL YEAR without my dad! Truthfully, I never thought that I'd survive without him. My dad was my absolute favourite person. My biggest fear after his initial diagnosis was that I truly wouldn't be able to go on without him.

But I'd done it. Everyone talks about getting through the first year—how all of the firsts are so hard—and here I was. I was practically fist pumping myself, because I thought I'd really crushed this grief thing!

I even had a conversation with a friend that Christmas morning exactly a year to almost the minute he'd died, and she congratulated me for making it through the first year. I watched her rub her hands together and say, "Now you can move on."

And that's what I thought was expected of me, but the truth is, I was sinking deeper into a thick, dense, mucky fog, oblivious to what was going on around me. On the inside I was torn up, battling so many extreme emotions while trying to cover up how I was truly feeling from the outside world.

2018 was the most difficult year of my life thus far, but it was also the year that I started a journey of healing and self-discovery that I never knew I needed or wanted, to be honest. When you're taken to the absolute depths of grief, self-loathing, shame, and despair, and then wake up one day and literally have it smack you in the face, it isn't that much fun.

The slow crawl back to a place where you feel whole, happy, grateful, and balanced again is extremely difficult. As I write this on the other side, I can truly say that I'm grateful for this whole experience—yes, even losing my Dad—which may be very hard to understand. But if he'd never left this earth, I would never have had to work through the things that had been holding me back in my life!

Hitting literally rock bottom started a path of growth which has ultimately made me a better, happier, and a much more confident woman, but the road getting here was long, dark, and had many twists and turns.

When I think about my life, I think of it in seasons:

Season #1: Dysfunctionally Perfect
Season #2: Controlled by Fear
Season #3: The Tipping Point
Season #4: Self-Awareness

Season #1 (the longest): My childhood and my teenage years, all the way up to my thirty-sixth birthday.

I coined it "Dysfunctionally Perfect" because from the outside—it looked perfect! Actually, up until "The Tipping Point," I thought it was perfect! I had a great life that so many people were envious of.

Of course there were little hiccups here and there, but nothing that caused me anything more than a few tears, and then life went back to normal, usually better than ever. From what I could see, everything was pretty status quo—in fact, way better than average!

However, so many things were happening, slipping by unnoticed (or so I thought), that would come back to haunt me in Season #3. They were all building up: the reason why I was so codependent, why I had such low self-esteem, and why the Tipping Point in 2018 was filled with so much built-up trauma that needed to be released.

Season #1 was a melting pot full of deep seeded dysfunction just waiting for the perfect time to boil over... which it most certainly did.

Season #2 Controlled by Fear

I was literally on high alert 24/7 for a full six years. When my phone rang, text notifications dinged, surprise emails came through, enduring the constant waiting for results, driving to and from hospitals... it was heavy—for two reasons!

My husband and I were smack dab in the middle of an adoption journey that would make any person feel extremely overwhelmed, and this perfectly coincided with my dad being diagnosed with Stage 4 Lung Cancer.

When we initially got the news of my dad's cancer, it was said in his words, "I have a little bit of cancer on my left lung. They're just going to slip in there, snip it off, and I'll be back at work in a few days."

Gotta love his positive outlook (one of the things I miss most about having him around), but unfortunately when they went in for the big grab—he was FULL! Full of cancer in all the wrong places, which led to no snipping at all.

He was stitched back together with all that cancer still safe and sound inside of him (I will never get that logic) and told that he was palliative, with eight months to live. This perfectly coincided with my husband and I having just gone through a second failed adoption. We'd been matched with a baby girl and on Day 30 of us being together, it fell through.

Both events were tragic and horrifying, but I handled it.

In fact, I remember specifically saying as we gathered in the hallway of the hospital, tears still staining my cheeks after hearing that my dad was palliative, that I was glad the adoption had fallen through. All I could think about was how I would get my dad better, and I declared that I'd never be able to be a good mother with this going on. Little did I know what was ahead, and how insensitive that sentence was to my husband, who was still reeling from our loss.

As an aside, this is not about my husband, Terry, but I have to say he is the REAL MVP in this story. Seriously, with what he's had to put up with, he deserves all the medals and MASSIVE love!

After getting the news about my dad, I went into an obsessive battle with Lung Cancer. I was having NO PART of him dying—100% NONE of IT! With the hours I put into researching lung cancer, you'd think I'd have cracked the code for curing it. I found every new test, exploratory treatment, surgery, anything and everything I knew and could quiz his oncologist about.

I was literally on a mission to save him, and nothing else mattered to me.

My dad pretty much tried everything to stay alive, even going through a radical surgery, as I mentioned earlier. He came so incredibly close to dying several times. No one can ever say he didn't FIGHT for his life like a CHAMP!

However, it was during these next few years that some family truths and discoveries would surface, and it was BRUTAL for me. I felt very responsible for keeping everything together for everyone else.

Somewhere in the middle of researching the latest cancer treatments our beautiful daughter came into our life. Delaney was the brightest and most amazing gift during all of this darkness. For me, though, the cloud of fear of losing my dad constantly battled my brain, and the burden and responsibility I felt for keeping it together was so heavy that it was hard to enjoy being a mom.

I know now that a lot of my shame would start to surface here.

I'd almost given up hope that I'd ever have the chance to be a mother, and when it finally did happen, I was so distracted I wasn't separating my own family (my husband and new baby) from my birth family (my parents).

It was confusing with everyone needing me. I truly thought I'd soldiered on beautifully, but looking back, I was a mess. It's hard to admit, but there's very little I remember about my daughter's first five years of life.

A few years ago I would have inserted a paragraph here saying something like t*his is no one's fault, I don't blame anyone, etc.*—trying to keep the peace and not hurt anyone's feelings. However, I'm not that person anymore.

I have a great relationship with my mom, and she is well aware of what I'm writing about. Because she's also such a huge advocate of personal growth, she's very supportive, and that's why I'm sharing some hard truths.

I was raised in an environment where it was expected—or so I thought—to pay more attention to other people's feelings than your own. Responsibility and "doing the right thing" or "being the mature one" were phrases that I heard over and over again. I haven't pinpointed if it was due to a need to "look a certain way" or if it was just a product of our family lineage and expectations.

What I now know for sure is that the way in which we are raised and the truths we are led to believe are all a product of how our parents, grandparents, and so on down the line were raised.

In some ways, I think we are all running around trying to figure out if we should believe and live in the way that we were raised, or if it is actually okay to believe and live in the way that feels right to us. It can be HELLA confusing.

At the end of the day, I think we are all somewhat of a big melting pot of dysfunction! And this particular season of my life brought out the dysfunction in a massive way.

Season #3—The Tipping Point

As I've told you, it was that one particular morning that everything surfaced for me. I looked into my eyes and knew that I no longer wanted to feel the way I was feeling. I felt beat up, battered, and internally bruised. My mind was so cluttered with sadness, anger, and resentment!

Grief seemed to be the catalyst that brought years' worth of shame and trauma to the surface. Memories surfaced that I'd stuffed deep down—things that scared me, and things that made me feel responsible for keeping our family together and happy.

The need for control and perfection consumed me. It also dredged up pieces of my personality that I truthfully wasn't aware were there—and it was ugly. I started a cycle of ugly comparison and lack of self-belief. Life felt so foggy that I truly didn't know what I was doing.

If you can imagine wrapping yourself up in thick cotton batting and looking out, that is what it felt like to be in my body. I couldn't see or hear anything clearly. I felt like I was a spinning top all of the time. Repetitive thoughts kept playing over and over in my head like a broken record, and they were all wrapped in anger, disbelief, and despair.

To cope, I became obsessed with my work in the most dangerous of ways; I was obsessed with being the best. I was obsessed with hitting the highest ranks, making the most money, looking a certain way, and doing it better than anyone else.

I was obsessed with doing GRIEF perfectly! I worked nonstop, ignored everyone in my life, and covered up all the hurt and ugliness boiling up inside of me with my hefty to-do list and business.

I got so caught up that I truly acted in ways that I'm certain hurt other people. I avoided people, cancelled get-togethers, and literally hid behind my computer for a few years — creating what I thought was a safety net that might somehow make all the pain disappear. I believed that I'd be able to outwork my pain and everything that grief had turned up inside of me.

I was very wrong. Looking back, this season would ultimately be the hardest thing to forgive myself for, and I knew that I should get help. My intuition kept saying *go talk to someone, Michelle*—but I refused to listen, so I just sunk deeper and deeper into this deep, dark place.

And then it hit. I caught my reflection in the mirror that fateful morning, and as the tears fell, I just knew that I couldn't go on like this for one more minute. I wanted out of this body, this suffocating bubble that I'd created. I couldn't breathe; my whole body was tingling, and I knew this was a do or die moment.

It was a moment in which you can literally see two paths in front of you. I knew if I kept heading down this direction that I would lose EVERYTHING! I'd already hurt so many people with my distance and decisions in the past few years, and if I continued acting like I was, I would lose the few that were still around, so I looked to the other path. I knew that I needed help. I knew that this wasn't going to be easy, but I could also see the LIGHT; there was light—and life again—ahead.

My inner wisdom guided me that morning. I am sure of it. She guided me out of the bathroom, right to my bookshelf. This was the moment that everything started to change.

Season #4—Self-Awareness

I walked toward my bookshelf. I had no idea why or what book I was going to grab. I was being directed solely by my intuition. I was nudged to pick up the book called *The Magic* by Rhonda Bryne.

I pulled it from its spot nestled between her other books, *The Secret* and *The Power,* backed toward my couch, and wrapped myself in a blanket while wiping away the last few tears. I felt so exhausted, but I knew that I was meant to open that book right then, and as I did I could smell the crisp new pages — and it started!

The book focused all around gratitude. It had a month-long challenge, with short tasks to do each day. I'm surprised that I didn't slam the book down, roll my eyes, ignoring the whole thing, because, honestly, what did I feel that I had to be grateful for at this point? Not much. But something pushed me, knowing that I had to start somewhere. I committed to the challenge.

As I flipped through the pages those first few days, as expected, my fear and ego (which I call my Inner Mean Girl) started appearing.

And she was fiercely trying to make me believe that I had absolutely nothing to be grateful for. She had me thinking this author—this stupid "woo woo" book—has no clue what I'm going through. But thankfully something made me keep going! I now know that it was my Inner Wisdom, who I've learned to tune into and trust, that kept nudging me to continue.

This truly was the first piece of the puzzle that helped me put myself back together—finding one small thing to be grateful for each day, even on my worst days. Each day it got easier. Even though I was still so confused and completely worn out, I could find little things to be grateful for each day.

My coffee, my workout, my house, the couch I was sitting on, my slippers, my daughter's smile, the one little giggle that snuck its way through the day before, my business achievements, the beautiful lake that we lived on... the point is: this book opened my eyes so that even on my darkest days, I could finally see the light! Even when you feel like you can't go on, when you're wrapped up in a cocoon of fog, light can peek through.

After I finished the thirty days, I felt a tiny bit of relief, and I was ready to see someone about the deeper issues that I knew were festering and were the reason why I was having such a hard time.

I made an appointment with a life coach, a woman I trusted very much. Now here is what I thought was going to happen: I'd share a bit with her, she'd give me some magic answers—a magic potion, if you will—and that would be that.

Similar to how my dad thought they would just snip out a bit of cancer, I was quite certain that was all I was going to need as well! And as you can imagine, I got similar treatment to what my dad did when they found more than just a wee bit of cancer on his left lung: she was having no part in "fixing me up," but she WOULD help me FIX MYSELF!

I'll never forget sharing EVERYTHING. It was the first time that I'd shared all of the truths, all of the things I had heard, seen, watched, and been a part of, which led to me feeling so angry, confused, and sad.

I unleashed the shame, guilt, fears—all of it—and she let me talk. I remember thinking, *my GOSH, just say something already, lady*...and at that exact moment she said, "You can't make me feel uncomfortable with your silence or your tears. I will sit here for hours until you feel like you've got it all out."

After what seemed like ages of me sniffling, wiping tears, not being able to talk, and then feeling like I'd talked too much, she gave me an assignment!

I thought *finally, here it is—this is what I'm paying for—the secret, the thing that will fix me up.* I was a bit shocked when she made me promise to set a timer for 30 minutes and WRITE, pen to paper, in a journal.

WHAT? She shared with me that this would be a pivotal part in my journey: getting everything I'd shared out on paper. It's not about pushing it away and pretending that it didn't happen; it's about acknowledging it and moving through it!

So I did it. And as I wrote, things got heavy, and hard. Tears fell, but just as quickly things started to feel lighter. Words changed. The force of my pen to the paper wasn't as heavy. By the end, I truly felt like 10,000 pounds had been lifted off my shoulders.

I truly felt like a layer of fog had been lifted. It was like I looked up and could see more clearly. It truly was the beginning of my healing. I was finally becoming aware, letting go of the past, letting go of my judgment, resentment, and anger.

I was finally seeing clearly again. That day started a massive journey of self-growth, an unraveling of moments, experiences, and a heck of a lot of forgiveness. I was forgiving myself for many things and also forgiving others.

From that day on, I've used gratitude, journaling, and silence (meditation) to work through what broke me open that day in 2018. Losing my dad was the catalyst that tossed my life around and surfaced trauma and pain that I'd shelved for so long and didn't realize was there.

On the outside looking in, my life looked fairly perfect. In fact, I am sure so many people reading this will almost find it unbelievable. I don't blame them. I felt the same, and that's why it took me years to uncover what truly had been holding me back for all of those years.

In the end, I want to leave you with a few lessons that I learned along this path to awareness that may help you if you find yourself in a similar situation.

1) ***Losing someone will be different for everyone.*** In our culture there are so many expectations and deadlines put on everything. This is what I have coined "Grief Judgement." Don't get caught up in that. Let yourself HEAL. Let yourself grieve. There are no magic timelines or ways of doing this. But from what I can see, you must work through it at some point, and I always think the sooner the better!

2) ***There is absolutely no SHAME in needing someone outside of your family or friends circle to help you process what you are going through.*** In fact, I now think that it's VITAL to get some help.

   Death is a trauma, and trauma will always uncover things that have been buried. That can be extremely confusing to navigate alone. Find someone who can help you process how you are feeling. Listen to your Inner Voice when it tells you that you need someone to walk you through this.

3) ***Forgiveness will SET you FREE.*** You may, like I did, uncover things that will need to be forgiven. You may need to forgive others, yourself, or both. This can be tricky when, often, the person you need to forgive is gone, or the person you need to forgive isn't someone that you feel you can speak with.

   This was the most pivotal forgiveness exercise that literally changed everything for me. I've shared this with so many of my clients, friends, and business partners since I learned it while listening to a podcast one morning a few years ago (again, the Universe gives you exactly what you need at the exact right time, if you're willing to listen).

Set up two chairs facing each other. Sit in one, envision the person you need to forgive in the other, and let it OUT... UNLEASH it all.

You can even switch chairs and pretend you are the other person. Hear what you need to hear, speak out loud what you would need them to say to you so that you can forgive them.

There is SO much power in forgiveness and it truly will change your life.

This book and every chapter in it is about HARD! Hard is subjective. Your hard and my hard may look extremely different.

If you are going through something hard, less judgment and more love toward yourself will help to set you free. If you know someone who is going through something hard, less judgment and more love from you will help to set them free.

Love is always a step in the direction of healing from the hard stuff... Like a Boss!

Chapter 10
NAZIA SHAHRIN

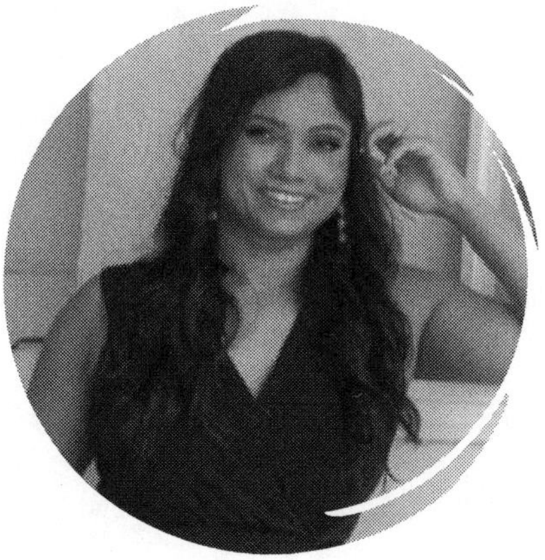

Photographer: Liz Salzman

Instagram @nazia.shahrin.to
https://ca.linkedin.com/in/nazia-shahrin-40935713

"Human beings are poor examiners, subject to superstition, bias, prejudice, and a PROFOUND tendency to see what they want to see rather than what is really there."

— M. Scott Peck

Introduction

The hardest things in life are not often the big, life-altering experiences that happen once in a while, but the small moments leading up to that big event that shape you. If you are about to go into war, it helps if you have fought battles before.

- The statistics speak for themselves. A recent government survey in the United States found:
- Women hold 14.6% of chair positions and 28.1% of directorships.
- Women represent 18.3% of CEOs and 32.5% of key management personnel.
- 30.2% of boards and governing bodies have no female directors. By contrast, only 0.4% had no male directors.

Almost half the population of the world is women, yet the corporate world doesn't reflect even close to that number after years of programs promoting women in leadership. If we are in the middle of a war for equality in the corporate world, why are women so behind?

It's the Little Things

"Wow, you actually have a proper technical degree."

This is not a statement that you expect to hear when you are interviewing for a technical leadership role, and while I was surprised, I also wasn't. The interviewer had already made some assumptions about me based on my gender even before I walked in.

"We are proud of the diversity we have built on this team."

I would hear that statement and look around to find myself being the only female in the room. The imbalance of women seems to be an invisible problem in many leadership rooms.

"Are you married? Do you have children?"

These are questions that have nothing to do with my ability to do a job but often seem to be a question I have to answer in interviews (I confirmed with my husband, who is also in technology, that he doesn't get asked these questions).

I realized that I had become desensitized over time to comments about women in technology and leadership. I now have standard answers to many of them and know that I have to spend some time getting the respect men naturally get when they start a new position.

Research shows that STEM fields are still struggling to keep women interested, especially in technology and engineering. Having spent the last 20 years in the technology industry, I realized the deterrents are not a few big challenges but a myriad of small experiences that a little girl or a woman faces throughout her lifetime that makes her question whether this path is really worth it.

To be successful in any path in life, we need a support system—a structure that shapes and builds our confidence and encourages us to keep going during tough times. As the African proverb states, "It takes a village to raise a child," and throughout time this village has been raising women very differently from men.

We are encouraged to be strong, yet follow a man's lead.

We are encouraged to be confident, but be passive in expressing it.

We are encouraged to lead like men but be a gentler, softer and less expressive version of them.

How is this related to what I, and many other female leaders, have experienced throughout our careers? Everything.

It started way back when...

> ***"Women belong in all places where decisions are being made. It shouldn't be that women are the exception."***
>
> *— Ruth Bader Ginsburg*

The reality is that women have not been a part of the forums where decisions were being made. History, also known as "His-Story," clearly depicts men as being the prime decision makers of all the world around us. We live in a world that was created by men, for men. This holds particularly true for the working world—especially the financial and technology sectors.

Women have been homemakers since the dawn of time. Men hunt, women raise children. What made sense hundreds and thousands of years ago shaped a culture that still looks at men as being the primary breadwinner and women being at home. The corporate culture has been built for men—the traits that are valued, the activities, the policies, and the behaviors all have a lens that speaks to men.

Over time this has become the norm for both men and women. When you imagine the CEO of a large financial institution, you see yourself imagining a man in a suit. Why? It's the same reason why you assume a child has a mom and a dad, as opposed to two moms or two dads. It has been the norm for so long that thinking otherwise does not naturally occur for us.

This normalization of what a leader looks and feels like—a very dominant, charming, extroverted man—has resulted in hiring and nurturing this bias. This is a form of implicit bias—where we find it easier to hire people we inherently feel comfortable with—and we feel most comfortable with people who remind us of our in-group, of ourselves. Lauren Rivera, an assistant professor of management and organizations at Northwestern University, spent two years interviewing people who were hiring entry-level candidates for several elite law, investment, and consulting firms. She found that although the companies did give considerable weight to education, grades, and capabilities, a heavy emphasis was put on "cultural fit." Cultural fit often meant things like sharing a common interest in certain sports or extracurricular activities or just being the type of person you'd be content to go on a business trip with. Now imagine this type of behavior in a technology firm, which is predominantly male. If the CEOs are almost all men for these companies, who are they likely to hire in their leadership roles? It really does start at the top.

It's a non-stop battle...

"You may encounter many defeats, but you must not be defeated. In fact, it may be necessary to encounter the defeats so you can know who you are, what you can rise from, and how you can still come out of it." -Maya Angelou

The journey to the top for women in the corporate world can be compared to pushing water uphill. At every critical step from the moment a little girl is born, she is shown a very different definition of success. Fairy tales tell little girls that her role in "Happily Ever After" is to find Prince Charming. The toys targeted for girls tell her being pretty and popular is what girls strive for. The worst of it is the unconscious and subtle ways society coaches little girls to be sweet, passive, and conforming, while teaching little boys to have no fear. We as a society teach little girls not to be risk-takers, not to be loud, and, most of all, not to be assertive, and to just get along.

This upbringing plays a critical role in the dynamics of a corporate world. It places women in an uncomfortable setting where the traits that were once applauded ensure that you are not heard in a room full of loud, confident men.

It doesn't just stop there. The upbringing allows others to intertwine your personal life with your professional life. Your relationship and marital status can easily become a blocker in your career, as the label "working mom" holds a very different connotation when opposed to "working dad." A "working dad" is just an employee; a "working mom" is an employee who has important responsibilities at home and needs "work-life" balance.

At every stage of a woman's life, she has to break the mold, challenge the labels, and confront the bias to be able to move a step forward. It's exhausting.

And it needs to stop... now.

"I tell my daughters to have their voice in this world, and it became clear I needed to role-model that."—Melinda Gates

We could spend years talking about the challenges that are holding women back in the corporate world, but I always tell my teams, "You have five minutes to get your frustrations out, then we work on a solution." That's what we need to focus on.

There are ways to change the culture in big, male-dominated corporations, and it will require women to step out of their comfort zones to make it happen.

Step 1: Authenticity

> ***"Be yourself, everyone else is taken."***
>
> *—Oscar Wilde*

When most of your week is spent working in an office, it makes a difference when you feel comfortable in your own skin. Being able to be your authentic self is something that makes a difference to your well-being and confidence. I am here as "myself" as opposed to who "they" want me to be. You are still moving the company vision forward, but you are doing it with your whole self. When women joined the corporate world, there was an enormous amount of pressure to fit in. You had to look the part and act the part. You had to change yourself so that others would be comfortable around you, as opposed to accepting you as you are.

I joined the workforce in the 2000s, and even then I was shocked when I had to have a conversation with a male mentor about the colors I wear to work. I was advised that neutrals are the way to go if I hope to be promoted. I always wear very professional attire, just in very bright colors. I am South Asian; we wear white for funerals and black is considered an unlucky color. I grew up seeing reds, yellows, and oranges, so they are what I lean towards. I listened the first time around and spent a year wearing grey, black, and navy to fit in. It mentally affected me. I felt like someone had stepped into my personal space. I rebelled when even my parents tried to tell me what to wear, yet here I was letting a man tell me what colors I should be wearing.

Then the big movement in tech started where everyone advocated to wear T-shirts and jeans to work. It was a movement to normalize comfort over the corporate look. Mark Zuckerberg wears T-shirts and jeans, and he created Facebook. During that movement, I went back to wearing colors again, thinking we are now more inclusive. And this time I was encouraged to wear jeans and casual clothes and give up my corporate attire completely so I would fit in.

That's when it dawned on me. This was not about the bright colors at all. This was about being different in a world where men set the standards. It's okay to bring your authentic self, as long as it fits the look and feel that has been set by the majority, which in this case was...men. T-shirts and jeans, okay. Crazy multi-colored socks—check. Orange and yellow dresses, no.

I had the opportunity to move to a female-led function later on in my career, where the ratio of leaders was close to 50/50 and I immediately experienced the difference in culture and tone. What I wore was never a point of discussion and there was an emphasis on embracing diversity. That is when it dawned on me: there was never anything wrong with what I wore. It was a lack of diversity in the function that led to a view that conforming to one way of dressing would set a positive cultural tone.

Trying to blend in with men in the office has not done women any favors. It has actually gone one of two ways: strong women become a shell of themselves to fit in, or strong women leave the company or role so that they can be themselves. Men are being themselves at work and have created the cultural norms even down to setting the norm for attire. If women are a part of this culture now, it's time that it evolves to be more inclusive of everyone. Be yourself, even if it does not fit the current culture. Eventually your authenticity will encourage others to bring their real selves to work.

Step 2: Network

> ***"I've always believed that one woman's success can only help another woman's success."***
>
> — *Gloria Vanderbilt*

One of the biggest advantages men have over women is the network and political currency they have built up over time in the industry. Women have joined the workforce later, and need to build this up for themselves and for others; to connect with people not just for their own progression, but to help progress others. The real change will come from lots of strong women in senior positions in many companies and sectors who will advocate for cultural change. You cannot do it alone.

When positions open up, even before the job is advertised, there are often discussions with people in the hiring manager's network to see if they know someone who would suit the role. This happens over casual conversations or even a simple ping to someone in that field to ask "Hey, do you know someone?" Women have been home makers for a very long time and are a minority in many high-performing sectors such as Finance and Technology. They are just not part of people's professional networks. The way to combat this is to put yourself out there. Even if you have a job, build a professional network in your field outside of your company. Men have built networks over professional engagements, golf games, and social gatherings for decades. Women have to be conscious of this and build theirs. Once you have a strong network, you will be the one they think of when a role opens up.

Step 3: Advocacy

> ***"I raise up my voice—not so I can shout but so that those without a voice can be heard. We cannot succeed when half of us are held back."***
>
> *—Malala Yousafzai*

For generations women have been taught to compete with each other. Female rivalry happens when a woman uses her power to keep another woman down, mistreats her, or competes unfairly. This goes back centuries to when it was about marrying the right man. Jane Austen's novels create a world that accurately depicts an environment where women compete and undermine each other for the chance to marry a wealthy suitor. While the corporate world may not be the same as an Austen novel, the coveted executive roles have replaced the wealthy suitors, and women often compete to be the few women in those roles.

My personal experience has shown me that there are women who pave the path for you and others who actively undermine your efforts to take you out of the running. It's not surprising that when you are so disadvantaged in the corporate world and so few roles will even consider you, the insecurity shapes your behaviors.

I never realized the importance of advocacy until I reached senior leadership. That was when I took a step back and recognized that there are some real systemic barriers for women. For example, almost all women I mentored struggled with career trajectory after having children. Many women struggled with voicing their opinion in meetings, as it would always be ignored and that was culturally accepted. The only way to change these big cultural and systemic problems was to have more women in critical roles of influence. The real solutions to the problems that need to be solved are beyond the one or two executive positions we want for ourselves, but to actually chip away at the cultural barriers that take women out of the executive pipeline in the first place. If we don't put mothers in senior roles, who will advocate for policies at that level to help support flexibility at the workplace for mothers? Who will make their male peers understand that a year of mat leave does in fact hurt your perception at work? In the end, it is a numbers game. One single executive cannot change the world. It will have to be a group of people who advocate for women's challenges in the workplace.

My biggest success at work has been the privilege of being in a position where I have been able to advocate for women to get promotions and take stretch-roles. In return, I have seen those women advocate for others, because when you are supported, that culture of competition fades and one of support begins. They have also helped me broaden my network in return. Advocating for others will not hurt your career, but will actually help you drive a bigger message to the top. There is strength in numbers.

Making Things Just a Little Easier

Everything we do for ourselves and women around us will help change the biases and assumptions for future women. Chances are, many of the changes will not be reflected until the next generation. Just from what we have seen in the news, black people are still fighting for equality and indigenous people in Canada are still trying to get everyone to understand what really happened in the past. Women are asking for a major shift in thought, and a change in cultural norms in large, well-oiled corporate engines that have thrived through decades and have made millions for shareholders. We are asking them to change their cultures to be more diverse, more inclusive, and to create equal opportunity and experiences for women. It will take time, it will take a lot of energy, and it will take a lot of investment in the three steps that I mentioned here to get rid of those little things that make career progression so hard for women.

> ***"Because I am a woman, I must make unusual efforts to succeed. If I fail, no one will say, 'She doesn't have what it takes.' They will say, 'Women don't have what it takes.'"***
>
> *— Clare Boothe Luce*

Chapter 11
NICOLE BELL

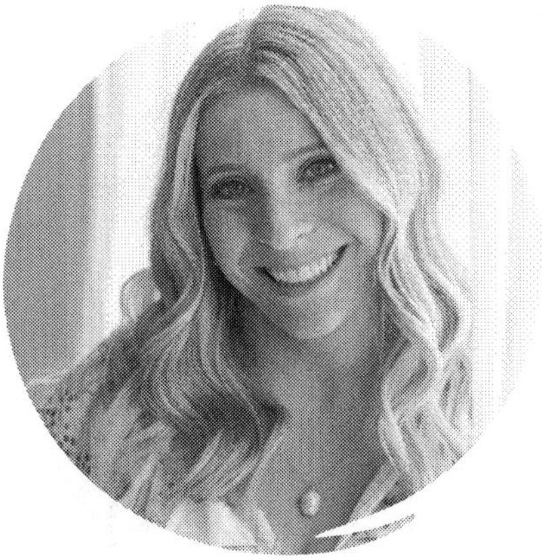

Photographer: Leah Smith

Instagram @nicolebell.wellness
www.nicolebellwellness.com

I was getting ready for a party on a May Sunday, sipping my coffee and listening to music. My phone chimed to alert me about a group text between my sisters, myself, and our dad. "I am in an ambulance on the way to the hospital. I couldn't get out of bed this morning. The paramedics said my glucose levels and others are very low, so they are taking me back to where I was last week." My stomach immediately sank because I knew that this time he probably wouldn't be leaving the hospital.

My mind started running in a million directions. We had been at his house the day before and he didn't look good. *I should have stayed the night with him...* I thought regretfully to myself. I should have actively forced him to go to the hospital like my sister had suggested. She kept asking him and we should have made him go. He looked awful yesterday, even worse than he did when he was in the hospital previously. He had barely eaten or moved during our visit, and complained about being freezing cold. I noticed that his jaundice seemed to have gotten worse. We should have never left him with her—his on again, off again girlfriend. We should have brought him home with us last night. What if that was our last visit with him, ever?

I rushed to wake my fiancé to let him know what had happened and to explain that he needed to get up and get ready. We were going to have to rush to the hospital in Barrie where he was being taken and it was well over an hour drive from us.

As we went through the motions of getting ready, my brain reeled in regret. I shouldn't have been so hard on him over the past two weeks. His girlfriend had said some horrible things to me while my dad was in the hospital the past week—that she didn't sign up to be a caregiver or to bury someone. Why hadn't I told her off? Why hadn't I believed my dad when he would talk about how awful she was to him? In the past, I figured if she had been so awful, why would he keep going back to her after every breakup? I just wasn't around enough to see all the signs—to see the signs that she, too, was an alcoholic and was far from able to help my dad. Whenever my dad would get sober and try to fight the awful disease that is alcoholism, she would just bring him down with her, leaving him again.

Over the better part of the last decade, my relationship with my dad had been rough. It hadn't always been that way. I grew up as Daddy's little girl, always looking for his approval and trying my best to make him proud. He introduced me to hockey and took me to my first Toronto Maple Leafs game the season the Air Canada Centre opened. He taught me how to ride a bike, how to be strong against all of my boy cousins, coached me during all of my years of playing competitive Ringette, showed me how to BBQ, how to drive the car and our boat, and showed us how playing outside is much better for our soul than sitting inside staring at a screen. He was a very present dad—the kind of fun dad who was always making it an adventure for us kids with the endless amount of yard toys he would purchase.

Our home had an open door policy; our parents always allowed us to have friends over and they made it a safe place. They were both incredibly social and some epic parties went down at 180 Daniels over the years. My childhood was fun and both of my parents were always there for me and my two sisters. I grew up knowing that I was lucky and feeling like I had it all.

My phone rang. It was my sister, who told me we should get ready, as they were on the way to pick us up. I've never had such an uneasy feeling in my life before. I felt like I was going to be sick. My sisters and our mom arrived, and we hopped in the car and immediately headed to Barrie. In the car I called my uncle, my dad's brother, to let him know what was going on. He and my aunt were up north at a friend's cottage. In a panic, he said they would leave immediately and get to the hospital as soon as they could. Next I called my aunt, my dad's sister. She immediately broke down, shocked by the news. They live close to Barrie, so she told me to give her a call once we arrived at the hospital. In the meantime, she would get her family together, including my Papa, who lives with them, to come to the hospital as well. I think I was in shock. *Is this actually happening today?* Were we *THAT* close to losing him?

Things hit a low in the summer of 2010. My parents were still together, but it was obvious that they were extremely unhappy. At this point there was no denying that my Dad was an alcoholic and that he had a huge problem. His skin and eyes started showing signs of jaundice for the first time, and whenever he drank none of us wanted to be around him. My sisters and I stayed out of the house as much as we could. I was 19 at the time, and as the oldest, I sat down to talk with my mom about everything. I couldn't take being around my dad when he was drunk any longer. All he would do was pick apart my mother. He would also turn on me, calling out my flaws, saying mean things, and embarrassing us when others were around. I told my mom that if something didn't change, I would take my sisters and leave. This wasn't a healthy environment for any of us. Later that week we all sat down with my dad. At first he was defensive and in denial, but then he broke apart. He agreed to stop drinking and go to the hospital to get a hold on his health.

My dad didn't have a family doctor. In fact, he rarely ever went. I don't really even remember him ever getting sick. At the hospital, he was first diagnosed with the beginnings of Stage 3 cirrhosis of the liver induced by alcoholism. He was given two blood transfusions, as his hemoglobin was so low at the time. The doctors didn't know how he was functioning normally. He was also put on medication for vasodilators to help improve his compromised liver function. He was referred to a family doctor as he needed to be under constant care. He was told that if he was able to stay sober that he could live with this for many years before needing a liver transplant.

At the time, he didn't tell us the actual diagnosis. He played it down to be less serious than it actually was, but we knew it was more serious than he was letting on based on his transfusion and the medication. At the time, I was in school to become a Massage Therapist. Most people don't realize the amount of physiology and pathology we learn. My best friend was in school for nursing, so between the two of us we understood that he wasn't being truthful. Unfortunately, that was a common trait for my dad during his struggle with alcoholism. He would lie all the time to avoid disappointing or upsetting people around him. Eventually it seemed even he believed his own lies. The problem was that he could never keep his stories straight, and we would always figure out the truth in the end.

He couldn't stay sober for long, and by early February 2012 my parents decided to separate. It was what they both needed. It was hard for me even though I was 20 years old, going to school, working, and about to be moving out of the only house I had ever lived in. I took it really hard and that was when I began to experience severe anxiety and panic attacks. I felt obligated to protect my sisters and to help my mom in any way I could. I became angry and resentful toward my dad—I didn't understand the disease of alcoholism as much as I thought. I couldn't fathom how he could choose drinking over his family, or why he was two different people depending on whether he was drunk or sober. I couldn't understand why he would make up such lies about my mom to our family and friends. I wanted to have sympathy for him, but I couldn't. I couldn't see past my anger at how he had single handedly flipped our lives upside down. Sadly, all of these are the effects an alcoholic has on those closest to them. Alcoholism affects the entire family, not just the alcoholic.

Things just got worse as the years went on. It was a rollercoaster, with highs and lows depending on whether my dad was sober or drinking. He never seemed to be able to go more than a few months of being sober before something would happen and he would spiral out again. He struggled to stay employed, which was shocking to us as he had been the hardest working man before. Even through the early years of his heavy drinking, his work was never affected. In fact, the only time he took time off was for Ringette or our two weeks of holidays in the summer at the trailer. Even then, his phone was still on and he always seemed to be on call. His depression took over every aspect of his life, and I no longer recognized the man I once admired as a little girl. I would get anxiety before seeing him and dread any family event with him. His behaviour was so unpredictable. He would say embarrassing or hurtful things to me, even in front of others, and I would be anxious for days leading up to a visit. My sisters and I started seeing him less. He'd cancel our visits together and cancel coming to dinner for our birthdays. Sometimes, it would be months before we'd see him even though we only lived 15 minutes from each other. That's when we knew he was drinking again; he would avoid us at all costs when he wasn't sober.

We arrived at the hospital and rushed in to find him in a private monitoring room right off of the ER, and the doctor pulled us aside immediately. He told us how low his blood pressure and heart rate were—that his glucose levels were in the range of a coma and that he was in an altered state from the toxins in his blood stream so we needed to prepare ourselves for that.

"How long? How long does he have? He was just released on

Wednesday from here saying he was stable and wasn't even supposed to see the liver specialist until a month from now!" My voice cracked trying to get the words out.

"It's unknown at this time how long he has. It could be today, tomorrow, or a few weeks from now. I've seen it all—but at this point I don't think there is anything we can do. So you are all okay to see him and just let me know his wishes." The doctor stumbled over his words. He didn't sound confident in a word he was saying. My sister is a Registered Nurse, so she started asking him a ton of questions about his levels, labs, and the treatment he had been receiving so far when he got admitted there. I tuned it all out. I knew she had it and would be best to deal with the doctor. My eyes shifted toward *her*, his on again/off again girlfriend, who was standing in the doorway to the treatment room crying. This angered me. One week ago she called me saying she was done and leaving him while he was in the hospital. Nevermind all the attitude, resentment, and lack of kindness she had toward my dad while we had been at the house just the day before. Little did she know that the night before, we had made plans with Dad to bring him home to live with us. We were going to come and get him that morning to bring him to our mom's house so that we could properly take care of him. He had agreed and was so grateful for it, but things went downhill very quickly for him overnight.

She hugged me while crying, saying how she just got here and told the doctor to discuss everything with his daughters once they arrived. All she knew was that it wasn't good. I was reeling over my anger at how this woman had treated my father. She couldn't even have rushed to be here with him. I decided to push past her and focus on my dad.

We went into the room and he was struggling to speak. We each said hello and gave him a hug and a kiss. He was so happy to see us all and my mom. He gave her an extra long hug. Before they separated and divorced, they had been married for almost 25 years. Although my mom hated the things he did, she didn't hate him and still had love for the father of her three daughters. Similarly, I never hated my dad, I was just angry at his actions and the things he had done in the past.

Even then, lying in the hospital bed, barely able to move, speak, or breathe, he was still putting on a front that he was okay. He cracked his typical kind of joke: "Man, they put a catheter into me this time, can you believe it?!" He chuckled. My sister asked him what he needed, and he said he was in pain and discomfort especially with breathing. We tried to adjust his positioning so he could breathe more comfortably. My sister then had to ask the hardest question she has probably ever asked in her life. "Dad, are you ready to go if something happens, or do you want to be saved?" He looked at her with tears in his eyes. "I'm not ready, save me please." My sister looked at me and shifted my gaze towards his catheter bag. It was full of blood. She grabbed my arm and dragged me into the hall. She broke down into my chest. I knew what it meant: Dad was bleeding out internally. This was the end, and most likely would be our last day with him.

I said "Okay, you go talk to the nurse and doctor, tell him he's not a DNR and get him something for the pain."

"Nicole," my sister's voice cracked. "They barely have him on anything right now, just glucose sugars. It's like they aren't even trying to help him! I don't understand!"

"Well you're the nurse, not me, so go talk to them. I'm gonna call everyone and make sure they get here ASAP!" I said, and sprung into action mode. Watching him like that, in that bed, with the death rattle breathing starting, made it hard to stay in there. I paced the hall of the hospital while I made the calls, finally breaking down to my uncle and aunt. I still couldn't believe we were there, even though deep down I had known this day was coming for a long time.

In the summer of 2014, my Dad hit rock bottom. When I thought he hit rock bottom in the past, it wasn't. That summer was truly the bottom. It was so bad that we held a family intervention with him, with his siblings pleading with him to go to an in-person rehab and that they would even deal with all the financials. He refused, but it was the first time I ever heard him say out loud, in front of me, that he was an alcoholic—that he had a problem—and opened up more about his mental health situation.

To this day, I believe that my dad was suffering from more than just depression; whether he had bipolar or borderline personality disorder, we will never know. My aunt got him in with a liver specialist in a hospital in downtown Toronto the next week. I went with him and the news was worse than he expected. His cirrhosis of the liver had changed to Stage 4 and there was very little viable tissue left. Being an alcoholic you have to be sober for over a year, be in a sobriety program like AA, and in constant care of doctors for his cirrhosis of the liver. The doctor gave him four years—at best—if he didn't take serious control of his health, and 7-10 years if he did, with the possibility of getting a liver transplant from a donor or a family member. The liver is the only organ in the human body that can regrow and heal itself. However, cirrhosis is the only thing that the liver cannot heal. The permanently scarred tissue cannot regenerate. I could tell that he was overwhelmed because he was quiet the whole car ride home. My heart ached for him, and I was terrified of the outcome.

Well there we were, almost five years later, losing my dad. His health was declining and he had kept it a secret for months. I think he knew it was coming because the past six months he had been sober, making good changes and behaving like the person I once knew a decade ago. We had really started working on mending our relationship. It was baby steps, but we were working on it. If I had known this was coming so soon, I would have tried harder to spend as much time as I could with him. Joe and I had gotten engaged that past February, and my dad attended our engagement party in March. Everyone commented on how much better he seemed and how it was like the old Steve again. He was so excited for the wedding and so happy to be around close family and friends. I wish he had told us what was really happening. It was selfish of him to keep this from us. Now he was dying and we had only known he was sick for a week. Maybe we could have helped him more? Maybe we could have pushed for better care at a better hospital? All of these maybes, all of these regrets, all of these could-haves and would-haves swirled around in my head.

My aunt, uncle, cousins, and Papa arrived at the hospital. I was so thankful they were here in time. By this point my dad could not speak, the "death rattle" breathing had gotten really bad, and he could barely keep his eyes open, but he saw his family arrive and I knew that he knew they were there. The energy in the room completely dropped. Those of us in the healthcare field knew this was it and that he was going to be gone within the next couple hours. My attention shifted towards my Papa, who seemed to be completely confused. He kept asking everyone about his prognosis. When he didn't like the answer that his son was going to pass away today, he asked the next person the same thing. He was still grieving over my Nana who had just passed away two years before. My heart shattered for him. Now we were all there, standing around this bed, and none of us were ready to lose him. It didn't matter about everything that had happened in the past, the pain that he caused, or the trauma that he put us all through. He was only 54 years old—much too young for this to be the end. Everything in the past disappears when you are standing there losing a loved one.

His breathing was getting extremely laboured and his stats were dropping. Since we had been there we never once saw the doctor again and a nurse only came in once. My sister started to panic. She was frustrated—we couldn't even find a nurse at the nursing desk. We wondered aloud, "Where the hell is everyone?!" My aunt called my uncle, her brother, to find out where he was. They had just parked and were rushing in.

I will never forget the sound the monitor made as all his vitals start dropping drastically. It's a loud, piercing, beeping sound that gets closer and closer together with red lights going off. My sisters and I rushed to his bed. My sister was holding his head whispering in his ear, "It's okay Daddy, you can go. It's okay to go." My other sister was holding his hand and I was standing right beside her. He flatlined.

My cousin ushered us back, thinking a crash team would probably rush in. But nobody came. A minute later a nurse walked in and shut the monitor off, followed by the ER doctor who checked his vitals manually and pronounced him dead. The room had burst with overwhelming emotion and tears. My uncle and aunt came running in—they saw us all and knew they were too late. My heart hurts for my uncle to this day not being able to say goodbye to his brother one last time. But in my soul I know my dad's spirit was still in that room and he was surrounded by his family, the ones who loved him the most.

There are many tough lessons throughout the grieving process, and even tougher lessons when it's the loss of a parent who suffered from alcoholism. The biggest lesson I have taken away from the loss of my father is that it is important to talk about it and not avoid the past. The more you bury the past during the grief, the longer it will take you to heal. It is natural when you first lose someone to keep replaying different events from the past in your mind. You can get caught up in the "would have, could have" moments and start to regret different things, but that won't change what happened. It happened and you cannot bring that person back to life. You need to give yourself grace and forgive yourself for any regrets you do have. It is very easy to look back on a situation and see the signs you missed. You might wish you had spent more time with that person, or wished you were a bit more kind, but you didn't know when you were going to lose that person and you did the best you could with the knowledge you had at that time.

Don't let anyone tell you how to grieve or the time you need to heal. This process is completely different for each person with the loss of a person so close to you. It is important to create boundaries to protect yourself during this time. This isn't selfish, but part of the grieving and healing process. Everyone handles grief differently and there are so many different ways that people can find peace with loss—and heal. Whatever way works the best for you, I encourage you to pursue, learn, and heal from your loss. Life is never easy, but when you can take a lesson from the difficult moments, that is the most authentic growth that you can go through in life.

Chapter 12
PEG CLELAND

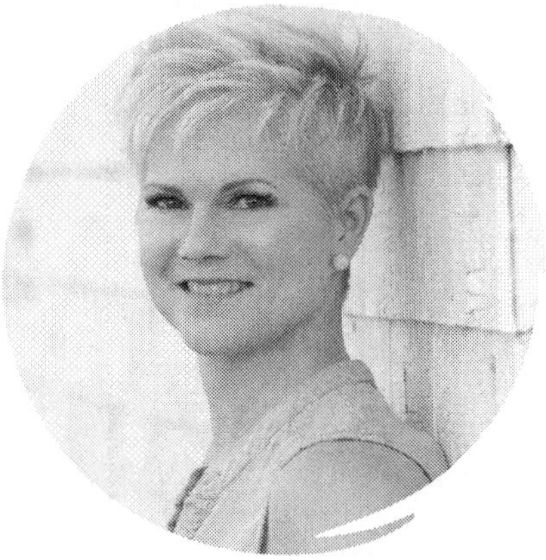

Photographer: Jen Talloden Photography

Instagram @pegclelandcoaching
Podcast: Between Your Ears
linktr.ee/PegCleland

Words. They hold so much power. And they can absolutely change everything.

We all know those 3 little words that change many relationships..."I love you."

My relationship was changed by 3 little words as well, but they were..."I am leaving."

That's how I found out my 22 year marriage was over. I'll never forget those seemingly simple words that came with so much complication in the shadows. It started with 3, but was followed by many other words that entered my mind during

those first few moments of impact. Words that would continue on replay in my head for hours, days, weeks, and let's be honest...years to follow.
How could this be happening to my 'perfect life'? This was never part of the plan. Not my plan anyway. But, it was happening, and in an instant my entire future changed and my entire past suddenly felt tainted and questionable...like it had all been one big fat lie. I was completely stunned. He might just as well have punched me in the face because that's how I felt. Barely conscious and not entirely sure this was real. But it was.

Obviously, I went through many emotions over the next few days, starting with disbelief, shock, and heartache, followed closely by frustration and resentment. Resentment when it really hit me that he got to make the decision. He decided what he wanted, and I didn't have any say. He got to choose and I had to live with it. He decided my future and I wasn't given an option.

That was 8 years ago, and I'm proud to say that after the initial shock, and all the shit that goes along with separating two lives and 27 years of 'togetherness', I *did* get to decide. We all have the power of choice in our lives. Maybe I didn't get to participate in the marriage decision, but I still had the power to choose what would happen next for me. The power to pick myself up and keep going. To decide on a new path for my future, and the future of my kids.

Oh those precious littles! To be honest, I know I gave them life, but they gave me life as well. What I went through in the days, weeks, months following the "I AM LEAVING" incident, was not nearly as important as protecting my kids. Ensuring they came through this whole situation as unscathed as possible, and that this complete change to our family dynamic didn't affect their sense of security or feelings of being loved.

I don't know how I would have gotten through this experience if I didn't have them. They were my reason to keep going. My reason to get back up as quickly as I could, and move forward. I guess that's my first tip. When your 'why' is big enough, you can do anything. When life gets hard, figure out what you want and why you want it. And I mean, figure out why you REALLY want it! Sometimes it will be staring you in the face and you'll know right away, but sometimes you need to dig beneath the surface to find it. Just keep digging until you find a 'why' that fuels you to keep going. Trust me, having a deeply personal reason to push through, will absolutely help you handle the tough stuff!

Now you know about my "hard thing", but before I share the good, the bad and the ugly of how I handled it, let me tell you a little bit about me. I am a single mom (you probably got that part) of two amazing humans, my son Keon was born in 2002 and my daughter Haley was born in 2004, the year I turned 40. I got started a bit late on my motherhood journey, and had some trouble with the process, but I always knew I was destined to be a mom! The slower timing turned out to be a blessing in disguise (thank you universe), because being 50 when my husband left, it was certainly nice to still have my kids in the nest and not be completely alone. My role as a mom/parent is truly my greatest blessing and the biggest, most rewarding, responsibility in my life...and I am pretty exceptional at it (if I do say so myself)!

Career wise, I taught school for 10 years before my love of health and wellness led me down the path of instructing, training, coaching, and "teaching" fitness. I believe I was born to be an educator. For years, I had the opportunity to travel the world in various roles within the fitness industry, and now I get to continue educating from closer to home, as an online thought leader and Life Coach. I focus on Mindset, Emotional

Intelligence. and the Human Design system in all of my group programs and 1:1 coaching sessions. My goal is to empower women and help them build self-confidence for their many roles in life and business. Recently, I launched a mindset and meditation Podcast called "Between Your Ears," so pop in your ear buds and come check it out! Even at my age, I am a growth junkie, so I will always be learning and then sharing my knowledge and experience with others (I also love a good glass of bubbly if you ever want to connect over cocktails!!)

Okay, back to the topic at hand. This next part of my story actually has a lot to do with my former career. My ex-husband and I lived a very entangled life and business. We spent over 20 years together, as a team in the fitness industry, and were often referred to as the Dynamic Duo. Yeah...not so dynamic, and certainly not a duo, anymore! Thus, our marital split was highly public and that definitely made things harder and even more a-w-k-w-a-r-d. We both taught classes at the same fitness facility (often as a team) and as you already know, this split was not something I saw coming...so I know it was just as shocking to our friends/members at the gym.

Even before word got out though (and sometimes that grapevine can be slower than you think), I made the decision to get back on the stage. Back to business as usual within the first few days. I kept telling myself, “just show up and pretend you’re okay”, because as I mentioned earlier, that’s all I could control... my choices. My decisions moving forward. To be honest, this was also partly a survival mechanism that kept me from curling up in the fetal position, feeling sorry for myself and hiding from the world. I can be a real introvert, so this hermit option was definitely tempting at the time. But, I think I knew it would only get harder and harder to face people, if I didn’t pick myself up quickly and move on. I pride myself on being resilient in other areas and past experiences in my life, this one just required a hell of a lot more effort to bounce back. I think there's a quote ..."the harder you fall, the higher you bounce". I was hoping for a big bounce!

Teaching fitness was also a welcome escape from the incessant thoughts in my head. Thoughts of past and future had no space between my ears when I was in the midst of coaching a class. Talking, cueing and moving in time to the music kept me in the present moment. Standing in front of a group of people, focused on coaching them, was a full-time distraction from the reality of my situation. Don't get me wrong, it was also an uplifting physical experience. We all know the endorphins that are released when we exercise, and trust me, I definitely needed those happy drugs! So there you go...a couple more lessons learned, and strategies I would highly recommend if you're going through something hard.

First, find ways to become present, so you're not constantly thinking about the past (which you can't change anyway) and the future (which won't happen unless you get out of the past). AND especially, so you don't miss the precious moments of living your life right NOW!

Second, boost your bounce-back, by moving your body... to move your energy! There are many benefits to moving, cleansing and releasing energy and emotions from our bodies. (Note: Yoga is very good for feelings of renewal and release, but punching a heavy bag can also be very 'therapeutic' when needed. You decide!)

Along with my kids giving me a reason, and my fitness classes giving me an outlet, I am also forever grateful to my family for giving me massive support to get through this challenging time. From holding me while I cried, to helping me pack up, move and get settled into a new home...they were always there for me.

And I know, this whole situation was hard for them too. They had all loved my ex over the years. After all, he was very likable and a pretty funny guy (but not nearly as funny after all of this!! Side note...I used to dream of tattooing ASSHOLE across his forehead, so everyone would know...and not be fooled by his funny guy routine!)

Okay, back to reality...

In the months and even years to come I often felt like I had let down the family's track record of perfection (we were the "Sunshine Family", after all, with no other divorces in the family album). I was the only one who moved away from our home city for a number of years, had my kids much later than my siblings, traveled the world doing crazy shit, and now, I was the only one with a failed marriage. It seemed like this was one more thing to make me a family misfit, and now I was the only one without my 'other half' at all family gatherings. Kinda like a 3rd wheel, 5th wheel...you get what I mean...the odd man out.

I now know this was *my* issue, and these were feelings of failure and disappointment that I placed on *myself*, but I think that's another lesson to consider. When other people are involved in your "hard things" in life...it can feel even more emotionally messy. Whatever you do, don't start making up stories that aren't true. Making things mean something they don't actually mean. Instead, talk to people about your feelings, get the story straight and stop carrying the burden alone. On the other hand, if you happen to be going through something on your own, and you experience negative emotions, give yourself grace. Be aware, be objective, and choose to make up a better version of the story for yourself...or simply LET IT GO (that Frozen girl was onto something there!). Sometimes you may even have to let certain *people* go. Be forgiving and gentle with yourself. Practice self-love. Take care of you...you're only human after all.

And as they say: "Shit happens"!

Speaking of shit, I'm going to take you back to the first few days after "the incident" because there's a lot to learn beneath that pile! Let's start with emotions, and there were many. As I mentioned, my first feelings were shock and disbelief, but after about a week things took a sharp turn down the path of complete anger. I'll never forget that Sunday morning, as the kids watched cartoons in the living room, oblivious to my mission of madness, I marched upstairs with a box of garbage bags and packed up all his shit in a matter of minutes. Of course it took a lot longer for me to pack up the emotional shit, but for now, all closets, drawers and cupboards were emptied of anything he didn't carefully place in his "I'm leaving" overnight bag. It felt good. Damn good, in fact! Like I was getting my revenge. Take that you asshole!! Obviously it didn't come close to evening up the score, but it was very satisfying in the moment!

I was tempted to throw it all away in the trash, just like he threw away our marriage. (See, I was definitely in the angry stage!) But instead, I chucked it all on the floor of the garage and sent him a sarcastic message, to come pick up his possessions (aka shit) at his earliest convenience. Even that felt too nice. At his convenience...again. His 'pick up' seemed far too easy. He made a clean getaway and I was left with the mess. Left to pick up the pieces of my life. Very inconvenient!

I used to think the stages of grief were reserved for mourning the loss of a loved one who died, but they really do apply to many situations in life, where we experience loss. Shortly after my 'wasband' left, my dad found an article about losing a partner and shared it with me (Dad was a very wise man, a wonderful teacher and I miss him dearly. His lessons and legacy will have to wait for my next book project.) The article talked about grief, and compared the feelings of loss between losing a partner to death, or losing a partner to adultery. It made so much sense to me. When a marriage ends because a partner dies, you lose your future with them, but you keep your past and all your shared memories. When a marriage ends because of a partner's infidelity, you still lose your future with them... but you also lose your past. You lose the purity of your memories. Everything seems tainted, like it was all a lie. You want to remove all signs of them from your life, instead of cherishing those old pictures on your shelves and photos in your albums. That's certainly how I felt in the initial stages of my grief. I wanted all signs of him GONE!

I also have to admit, as terrible as it sounds, I momentarily wondered "what if". What if he had been hit by a bus the day before? What if I never heard those words "I am leaving."? What if I didn't know he stopped loving me and had secretly found someone else? How would my life be different? How would I be different? But those were questions not worth wondering about. Not worth searching for the answers to, because that was not my reality.

Later (much later after I worked through all my stages) I was able to acknowledge that my ex-husband and I did have a number of great years together, we did support each other's growth, we had some wonderful adventures as a couple and most importantly...we created our two amazing children. So, I will always be grateful that he was in my life for a season...and a very important reason!

This brings me to another lesson I learned during that time in my life. It's from a chapter in the book *Think and Grow Rich*. The book is not specifically about money...but rather, about growing a rich life. It suggests that every time something negative happens in your life, you should search for 3 positives that were a result of that situation or event. This lesson has stuck with me in many areas of my life since then, but with respect to my husband leaving, these are the positives:

1. I decided to be present in every aspect of my kids' lives. Of course I would have 'basically' done this anyway, but I'm sure I would have missed some things because my husband could go to the game or take them tobogganing etc, while I got some work done, or tidied up the house, or any number of other meaningless tasks. When you have a partner you can split the load, and I realize that sometimes that's necessary. BUT, when you have no one to tell you how the game went, or when your child did something outstanding...then you better show up yourself! Time goes by so fast, and I decided not to miss a thing! Every game, every event, every opportunity to be there and support them. And now, my relationship with my kids, who are 18 and 20 is absolutely amazing! I know this was a real positive for us in the long run.

2. I learned to trust myself with money. That had always been one part of the marriage I left up to him...the finances (even though I was the bigger income earner for most of our marriage!). Suddenly, I had to learn all "the stuff" involved with the bank, bills, mortgage, car payments, investments, etc...and it felt like a lot in the beginning, but as time went on it gave me a real sense of independence and I was proud that I could handle it all.

3. I learned that communication is everything! Of course, it was too late to turn this around for my marriage, but I share this lesson with many married friends and I also apply it in all areas of my life, especially with my kids. We humans can't read minds (at least not yet!), and many relationships in our lives would benefit from more communication and less assumption! Less assuming that

> you know what they're thinking, or you know what's going on, and more listening and asking questions with the intent to understand. I encourage you to actually talk with your partners, making eye contact and everything! We can go through our daily lives thinking we've had conversations with our loved ones, but truly it's just been passing thoughts and surface exchanges. There are so many distractions in our world these days and we're losing our ability to focus. Commit to being 110% present if you truly want to build a deeper connection... with anyone! Your partner, your friends or your children!

These 3 lessons, and this entire exercise of reframing events in our lives is not always easy. Some situations seem completely negative and dark until you sit with them for a while. Eventually, we can always find something positive...rising out of the ashes, so to speak. I encourage you to give it a try in your life, and remember this quote as well..."Life doesn't happen to you, it happens *for* you." How can you see an event from this perspective? How can you see a negative situation as something that is offering you an opportunity for growth, learning and perhaps, a positive change?

Life does happen for us. I know this to be true. So many blessings have come into my life because of this one hard thing that happened TO ME. This one hard thing that happened FOR ME!

Hard things often alter the trajectory of our lives. That one incident that shifts everything and we start moving in a completely different direction...which reminds me of one of my favorite movies. Have you ever seen *Sliding Doors*? If not, I'll give you the basic premise behind the story. Gwyneth Paltrow's character starts the movie as one character, but after a certain incident occurs....the storyline shows us two separate pathways that her life could potentially follow. Two very different outcomes, impacted by one moment in time, that determined her future.

I often see my situation as just such a moment. Time stood still when I heard those words "I am leaving", and then my alternate pathway emerged. My future continued...just in a slightly different direction. I felt cheated in the beginning, like my perfectly planned route had been erased from the map, but after years of living this new path, I can honestly say that I love this version of my story. My relationship with my kids, my trust in myself, my growth as a parent, my independence as a woman.

I now have no regrets, no what ifs...only gratitude, trust and celebration that this was the journey I was meant to take. I hope in some way my story and lessons have been helpful. I hope they support you in navigating your own relationships, break ups, parenting, comebacks and all the other stuff that's part of this great adventure called life.

I said at the beginning of my chapter that words are powerful. They hold a great deal of emotion and meaning for each of us. Words can change everything, and now, these are some of my favorite words:

I am okay.

I am enough.

I am an exceptional mom.

I love my life.

I can handle hard stuff!!

Chapter 13
SHARANA ALI

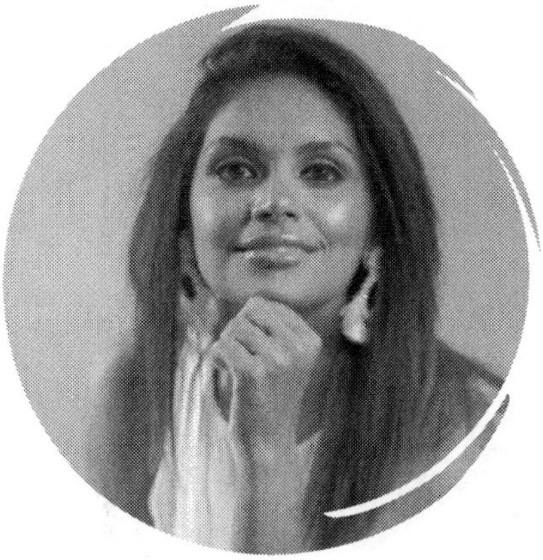

Photographer: Liz Salzman

Instagram @BOSSTheSixEdition
Bossthesixedition@gmail.com

I grew up in the 90s. I mean, I was born in the late 80s, but what do you actually remember from the first couple of years of your life? For me, not much at all.

My earliest memories were probably around grade 2, so I was 7ish—and already, the seed was planted.

Before we go further—MAJOR TRIGGER WARNING—I'm flashing lights here, sounding alarms, and shouting from the rooftop. I'm talking weight loss, negative body image, body dysmorphia, and bulimia. I'm about to get down and dirty in an effort to show you how I went from desiring to take up no space, to living a life where I want to live LOUD and TAKE UP ALL THE SPACE.

Weight Watchers, Jenny Craig, Richard Simmons, SlimFast, and that dreaded cabbage soup diet were in their prime in the 90s. "The Big 5"—Naomi Campbell, Cindy Crawford, Linda Evangelista, Christy Turlington, and Claudia Schiffer graced the front cover of every magazine. While most seven year olds were downing dunkaroos or slurping Fruit Loops as they watched Pinky and the Brain, I wanted nothing more than to look like the popular, beautiful, Kelly Kapowski with her long luscious hair, pencil thin waist, and, of course having the eye of the most popular guy in school.

Taking up as little physical space as possible was "the" thing at that time, and while that's certainly not new to the 90s and a little curt around the concept of dieting—at seven, what difference did I know?! In my adolescent mind it boiled down to a simple equation: be skinny = be cool = acceptance. At seven. In a world that didn't even know social media. Now, as an adult who has had, and continues to work through, this mindset, can we all agree: HOW SCARY FOR A YOUNG MIND?!

I'm Sharana Ali; you can often find me slaying the mean streets of downtown Toronto as an employee of the Ontario Government, or owning my beautiful world of BOSS (Brunch Opportunity and Support System), a business stemming from the concept of speaking your truth over brunch. More importantly, I'm a single mom on a mission to normalize what it looks and feels like to be the parent you always dreamed of being, on your own terms... even through the meltdowns (yes, for mom and kid). I'm 30-something, proud at 5 feet tall, often fluctuating between 110-140 lbs. Only now can I own the beautiful truth that none of the above defines who I am as a person. Especially my weight. I only realized this in my 30s! That's only a few years ago. And while it's never too late, I would do anything to change the narrative for people—particularly women.

It wasn't until very recently that I could look at myself in the mirror, and smile. It's only now that I realize that the worth of my existence isn't in the numbers on the scale, the size of the dress I wear, or the ratio between my hips-thighs-breast, because the truth is that no one gives a shit—and therefore, I shouldn't either. The "fun" part of this is that I didn't just wake up one day and say "hey, let's just love this body." It's a choice... daily. Sometimes hourly.

As I move through my day, it often means reminding myself that I can eat whatever I want. I can wear whatever I want. I don't have to "punish" my body for looking a certain way. I don't have to work out until my body is too sore to move, or search for a magic number just to leave my mark on this world. And on the days when I feel like binge eating pizza while watching *Friends* for the millionth time, IT'S OKAY. It is ALL okay. Because the truth is (and I found this out the hard way), no one will love you the way that you want to be loved unless you love yourself that way.

Today, I know my body IS my story. The way it curves and contours; every mark, line, fold, dimple, pimple, scratch, and scar. It's mine, and it tells a tale of love, adventure, pain, and mystery. And if I could go back and speak with that seven-year-old me, I would look her in her eye and tell her: you are so god damn beautiful as you are; show the fuck up and be proud of what you bring to this table, even though it feels like this world isn't for girls who look like you. It is for you—make it FOR YOU.

How the hell did I get here? How did I go from marking my "Precious Moments" calendar that hung in my lavender childhood room everytime I threw up—to now, trusting my body and its power? Honestly, I had a daughter. I needed to be a role model and realized that I couldn't preach loving yourself and living your best life if I hated who I was and what my body looked like. I needed to walk the talk out of fear of being called out as an imposter.

Before the first steps of that journey toward realizing my power had nothing to do with my physical stance; the goal was always zero. I wanted to be a size zero. Nothingness. An extra small. As little as I could get, to take up the least amount of physical space as possible; and if that meant withering away to nothingness...Sign.me.up.

I never wanted to toy with my health. I was "smarter" than that. I never wanted to jeopardize my lush hair, or strong bones; but my actions came at a cost. My body was the one thing that I felt I could control; if I could just train my mind and body to discard food—I, in effect, would be more digestible.

By taking up less physical space, I would be a more palatable person. People would accept me more; I would be seen as pretty, as a good girl, as worthy, as "girlfriend material," as sexy, as employable. What I didn't realize at the time is the message of being small that I constantly reminded myself of, was so much more than just keeping my body small. It was keeping my presence small, my ideas small, my goals and successes small—ultimately for the acceptance of those around me.

I would often scan my body from a very young age (Grade 2), noticing the differences between myself and those of the bodies that I saw as "beautiful." I would hear my mom talking about Jenny Craig, or picking up a bottle of Slim Fast to lose a couple of pounds. While weight was never an explicit topic in my household, it was always understood (or maybe assumed by me) that as a little girl, the quieter, smaller, and less space you take up, the "cuter," more digestible, and acceptable you are. And so, at such a young age, I understood that if I wanted to be smaller, I needed to consume less—or get rid of whatever I consumed. And so I did.

It was simple math; what went in must come out. If I ate 100 calories, I need to rid myself (however possible) or at least 150 calories. And so each night, after dinner, I would head to my room to have a shower and prepare for bed. Reminder, I was seven. Just like my body was still growing, my mind was, too, and I was extremely malleable to wanting to do whatever it took, to be noticed. As I would turn on the shower, in our family shared home with 1 full bathroom; I would prepare my toothbrush. This, at the time, was my weapon of choice. While showering, I would make myself throw up. Mentally, I was able to justify it all. The food is no longer in me, it couldn't add weight to my then 120 pound frame. I remember washing the vomit down, with such pride. I did it. I was serving myself. And, as I would return to my room I remember marking an "x" on my calendar for each day, and each time I would throw up.

It was my reward. Like a child's reward chart, after a certain amount of "X's" I earned something. Except, there were never enough "X's". There was no reward at the end. Truthfully, I wasn't losing weight at all—but still, I felt in control. I felt like I was working toward some ultimate goal.

In grade 4, the journey to worthiness took form through starvation. I would eat a small breakfast (I had to before leaving home), skip lunch, no snacks, and after dinner - I needed to earn that X; and after a month of X's ... instead of skipping lunch, I would eat an entire KitKat—200 calories, no problem. I hadn't eaten all day, I deserved it.

In highschool, it meant skipping lunch and a small dinner without carbs. Never any carbs. As though a piece of bread or some pasta was what was 'making me fat'. Food was the enemy, and it was my duty to do whatever it took to ensure it did not win this fight.

In university, I was on my own. THIS was it, this was the moment I craved; I controlled what I could consume - I controlled how often I exercised, and you would think; with the warped mindset I had carried to this date, I would somehow spiral out of control. I didn't. In fact, in my second year of university, I hit my highest weight. I was disgusted with myself, couldn't believe my lack of self control; only now to realize, while I saw food as a hurdle, I was using it now as a method of comfort. Eating, to fill gaps of being away from home; eating, to sustain long nights of studying and partying harder than I'd like to admit. Until one day, I stepped on the scale, nearing a "fearful" 150lbs on my 5 foot frame, I had enough.

The exercising - starvation cycle began, except a new player had entered the game. Laxatives. After a heavy meal, or anything I deemed indulgent—I would take a few. In no time, I was sick to my stomach and glued to the toilet for hours. It was physically painful, mentally—I had convinced myself, I was going what needed to get done. While I lost a few pounds, it was never enough. There was always this deep rooted fear in me. If I was too big (whatever, that meant) - I wouldn't be pretty enough, my then boyfriend would leave me, I would be alone - ugly and unacceptable; never being able to live a life I dreamed of.

As I neared my mid-20s life began to change, I was working now - hanging on tight to the promises of green tea, popping apple cider pills like it was my morning vitamin (I convinced my parents I needed to take these to 'help with digestion'), working out daily and treating myself with the allowance to 1 double double coffee a day. Breakfast - hah! Who needed that?! Lunch, a salad ... GET AWAY FROM ME grains! Dinner, well, I would throw it up anyways . There was great shame in my ways, no one knew what was happening, no one could tell. I didn't 'look' like I had disordered eating—in fact, I looked like any other girl who's weight would fluctuate.

I began to live the dream - good job, married, condo downtown Toronto - for so many, it seemed picture perfect. And still, the folds of my stomach - and touching of my thighs reigned above it all. I continued to convince myself; I wasn't sexy. I didn't deserve this. And, if I didn't keep exercising and looking a particular way, I would loose it all.

The negative internal conversations were continuous; no one outside of my mind knew what was happening. I felt like a sleath con artist, getting away with a crime that now as I look back was only harming myself. But ultimately, WHY?—why did I want this so bad? How was I convinced this would better my life.

Honestly, now in my 30's I still don't know. And the truth is the cycle continues to this day. I don't starve myself today (actually, I've built an entire business around across the greater Toronto area); I don't count calories - but I do make the conscious decision each and every single day, to no longer allow myself to slide down that slippery slope.

And why, because I got pregnant.

With the flash of a plus sign, I was responsible for something larger than just me. I now needed to set the tone for what I wanted for this little human. I needed to change my narrative, internally and externally to ensure that I was equipping this little human with the chance to thrive and truly believe in their power. I needed to walk the talk, so that one day, those little eyes couldn't turn to me and call me a hypocrite. More than that, I wanted better for us both. I wanted to get healthy. I wanted to take control of my life, as a commitment to us both.

I wish I could say, I saw the value in me to say the 'switch flipped'. It had nothing to do with me, yet everything to do for me. I started trusting my body, listening to its cues and placing worth in its power for her. It was so one day, she would know that she is as powerful as they come. She could confidently say, that she saw her mom be proud and stand tall in her essence, instead of hiding behind what society told her she needed to look life.

Five years of motherhood will test you. Especially when it comes to your body. Especially, when once upon a time its worth and value was placed on being 'flawless' and as small as possible. For nine months, I slowly and steadily expanded—proud of my tiny bump, excited as I saw the scale climb but still conscious 'not to gain too much weight'.

It is and was a constant mind game. A circus of thoughts, met with ultimately choosing myself daily. And in the choice, it's the promise to be healthy, to change the language I use towards myself and amongst the circles I partake in. Ultimately, I don't know if I come out looking like a BOSS daily, but I certainly feel like a BOSS.

I feel like I am finally happy. I feel like I am finally in a good place, where the choice to make healthy choices comes a little easier. It means, no longer depriving myself, but instead realizing and sitting in the fact that I am worthy far beyond the number on the scale, the amount of "x's" I had on that precious moments calendar, beyond the size of my clothes but instead on how deep I laugh, how bold I take chances and more than anything else, how I show up for my daughter.

Chapter 14
TAAHIRAH ISSANY

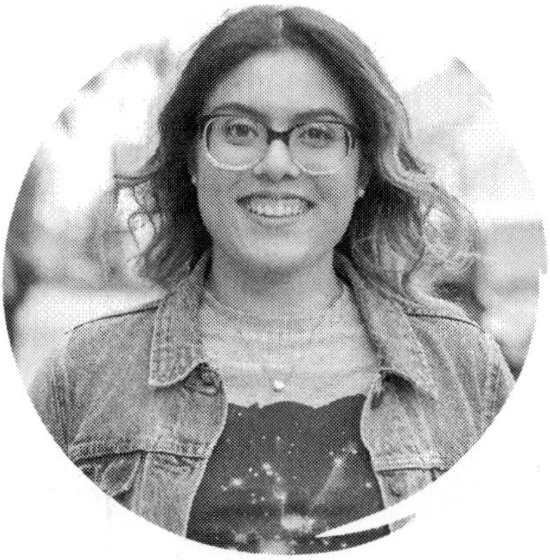

Photographer: Photography by Azra

Instagram @taahi87

Your family doctor said that we could introduce solids at four months old, but we waited until just after six months to start. I could tell that you were ready earlier; all of the signs were there, but in all honesty, I wasn't ready. Whenever I thought about it, a sense of dread crept over me. What foods do I start with? What should I avoid? What foods would you like? Would you have a sweet tooth like your mama, or like more savoury things like your dad? I kept on thinking about the mechanics of how humans eat. How was a baby supposed to innately know what to do when food is put in their mouth? I mean, you were a smart baby, Sophia, but how was your natural instinct supposed to tell you when you needed to chew, how to swallow, and when to swallow? There was no way that I could teach you this when I struggled to swallow myself. My body didn't seem to have that natural instinct that most humans do, so maybe yours wouldn't either.

Your first food was broccoli. Don't ask me why we thought it was the best thing to start with.

The minute you took a bite, the gagging commenced and I couldn't handle it. Nothing can prepare you for when a baby starts to gag. I stood up and my heart was racing. I felt helpless. I couldn't teach you how to do this. It's something you would have to learn on your own. I decided that perhaps you weren't ready. We'd try again another time, I said to myself.

Later that night, as I thought more about it, flashbacks of all of the times that I struggled to eat food came flooding in. The excruciating chest pain from the food that wouldn't go down, my eyes watering from the discomfort, the run to the bathroom when my body decided it was rejecting the food that I had swallowed. You starting solids was more triggering than I had realized it would be, but I knew that I needed to get over the anxiety quickly because I didn't want my fears to be projected onto you. My daughter would not be a picky eater like me.

Granted, I had my reasons for being this way, but you would not follow in my footsteps. I would not let that happen. You would understand why mommy couldn't eat certain things, why she had to step away from the dinner table sometimes, and why she always drank hot water. But how would I explain everything? I've always avoided talking about this with other people, but you deserve to hear what your mom has gone through—the good and the bad—and what I've learned (and am still learning) from it. Some good has to come of it.

I have always felt that when I tell my story, people will look at me differently—that they will just see my illness. That the person they knew before will be erased. That Taahirah Issany, the mom, the traveler, the accountant, the lover of a great french pastry, will be overshadowed by the decade of my life that I spent not knowing what was wrong with me. But I've come to learn that while I still live with this illness every day, I cannot let it define me. I've taken back the reins and it no longer controls my life. Instead, I've let it become my little shadow that follows me wherever I go, but it will not rule my life like it did for so long.

It started when I was in grade seven. I wish I could remember the first time it happened, but all I do remember is that I started hating bananas. I just found them difficult to eat and I had no idea why. Then the difficulty progressed to other foods at various times. I had to excuse myself on a number of occasions at the dinner table and run to the bathroom because the food I swallowed was in limbo. It didn't want to go down and there was nowhere else for it to go but up. When my mother tried to talk to me about what was happening I shut down. I didn't want to talk about it. I didn't want to try and describe to her what I was feeling because it was like reliving it all over again. Not just that, but it was hard for me as a then 12-year-old—still a child—to articulate exactly what I was experiencing. I just couldn't describe it in enough detail. I just knew that I couldn't eat things and I didn't know why.

Your grandmother was worried, so she did what every parent would do: she brought me to the doctor. I went to one of the best Children's hospitals in Canada and they ran various tests. They first diagnosed me with GERD (which I have come to learn is a common misdiagnosis) and gave me some acid reflux medication. Both my parents and I were hopeful. I took the medication as prescribed, and sadly my symptoms persisted. It wasn't GERD. We were disappointed, but we still had faith that they would figure out what was wrong. I was poked and prodded again, diagnosed with something else, and the cycle repeated, until they ran out of diagnoses. With every misdiagnosis and visit back to the hospital, I was a little less hopeful and a little more skeptical of my doctors, until I lost complete trust in the system that was supposed to help me.

When the possibilities were exhausted (in their opinion), my doctors concluded that it had to be in my head and they sent me to go talk to someone. Mental health issues were not something that were as commonly talked about then as they are now, so I was confused as to why they thought this was the best course of action. Looking back, I realize what they were trying to imply but were perhaps too afraid to ask me outright. They thought I had an eating disorder. Now, if they had just observed one of my episodes, tried to watch me eat something, seen me struggle so hard to do something as simple as swallow, they would have never gone down this path. They would have seen that I wasn't voluntarily throwing up, but rather it was something that my body was doing on its own.

When the mental health care professional concluded that I exhibited no signs of an eating disorder, I gave up. I went to a world-renowned hospital—if they couldn't figure out what was wrong with me, who else could? I didn't want to feel like a lab rat anymore, being poked and prodded only to be told there were no answers. I wanted to feel like a teenager again and start high school like a "normal" person. Little did I know, that was never meant to be.

As I started high school, my symptoms got worse. What used to be a struggle a few times a week became a daily struggle. I would have problems eating at least one meal during the day. The feeling of having food stuck in my throat came more often, only going away after drinking water or having to vomit. As these instances became more frequent, so did my anxiety. I couldn't predict when these "episodes" would happen, so then

I became fearful of eating food. There was no rhyme or reason (or at least none that I could figure out) as to what my body would or wouldn't accept to be swallowed. One day it would allow ice cream and the next day it wouldn't. I became fearful of eating in public and I started going out less and less, becoming more shy and more of a homebody. I didn't want to end up in a situation where I'd have to explain why I didn't want to eat food, or worse, explain one of my episodes. How do you explain something that doctors haven't been able to explain? Would anyone believe me? I worried that people, as many had, would assume that I had an eating disorder and make judgements about me based on those assumptions.

Teenagers can be mean and high school was difficult as it was, so I learned ways to hide it in public. In social settings I would commonly say "oh, I just ate," or "I'm not that hungry." A classic tactic would be to share something with somebody at a restaurant and just let that person eat most of the meal. You never really understand how integral food is to social interactions until you can't eat at them, but it was the cause of so much of my anxiety. None of my friends noticed anything wrong. I was losing weight but nobody really noticed because I grew a lot during this period and they just assumed it was puberty. It was easy to camouflage my pain back then.

When I started university, my symptoms worsened further. I had difficulty swallowing most things. Every meal I would have to run to the bathroom. I was afraid of all food, even the ones that I used to love eating. I retracted further into myself. I played it off as keeping busy. I worked multiple jobs through university so that I had "no time" to socialize. I was a shell of my former self, just trying to get by and make it to the next day. I began to think about my own death; not suicidal thoughts, but more so I came to terms with the fact that this thing—whatever it was—was probably going to kill me. I still didn't want to know what it was, though. I was still too afraid to face the monster.

When I graduated and started working full time at an accounting firm, the coughing started. I began to have trouble sleeping, and swallowing liquids now too became a challenge. People started noticing something was up and I couldn't hide it as well anymore. It started affecting my performance at work. The turning point was when I had lunch with a partner at the firm I was working at. It was the salmon that got me. Why did I order the salmon? It was always so hit and miss for me. We were having a casual lunch to discuss my performance, and from the first bite I knew I was in trouble. I had no alternative but to continue to pretend to eat while trying to make small talk. With every bite the heaviness in my esophagus grew, and I knew this would not end nicely for me. I tried all the normal tactics to help get the food down, but they proved ineffective. Instead of flowing conversation my responses became short, "mhmm" and "ahas" until my body decided it had had enough and I had to run to the bathroom, cutting my partner's evaluation of me short. When I returned, I apologized profusely, saying I felt ill: "it must be bad salmon." I couldn't tell him the truth—I didn't even know what the truth was myself.

From that point something changed in me. I woke up. Instead of being afraid of what this illness could be, I needed to know what it was. I was ready to face the monster. Up until that point I had wanted to live in oblivion, fearing that the prognosis wouldn't be good, there wasn't anything that could be done, or that it would be terminal. The fear of death had been all-consuming and crippling, and one of the main reasons that I never looked further for answers about my illness. I had been telling myself that I was too young to die; I had so much life to live. But what kind of life had I been living? I had been too scared of what might happen to do much of anything, so what was the point of living like this anymore? I thought I couldn't handle the truth, but enough was enough. If I was going to die, I at least wanted to know what I was dying of.

As an adult I was referred to a different specialist. I was skeptical, of course. She told me the tests she wanted to run, which happened to be the same tests that I had done when I was a child. I remember the first test, the barium swallow. As I was attempting to down a liquid that tasted like chalk I was thinking to myself, *what were they going to see now that they didn't see back then?* But by then it was too obvious to ignore—even the technician who was performing the test could see it. "Achalasia," he said. "Aka -excuse me?" I said. I had never heard of it. But a simple Google search told me all that I needed to know.

Achalasia is a rare disorder—in fact, most doctors won't come across it in their lifetime. It occurs when the muscles at the end of the esophagus (which are used to push down food) become damaged somehow and it becomes difficult for it to push food down to the stomach. My doctor told me that in my case it had become so bad that gravity was the only thing that was getting my food down - my esophagus had essentially given up.

The list of symptoms fit mine: trouble swallowing, chest pain, coughing, vomiting, weight loss, and heartburn, although they varied from person to person—which often led to misdiagnosis.

Prognosis—incurable, but surgery could help alleviate symptoms. Not the greatest news, but any help to ease my symptoms would help.

Cause—unknown. *Great,* I thought to myself. I didn't even have something/someone to blame for getting this.

Surgery was my only course of treatment, but I was cynical. How was punching a bunch of holes in my esophagus supposed to make it work again? Were we going to poke it until it realized it had been sleeping on the job for a decade? I had hoped speaking to the surgeon would alleviate my skepticism and revive my faith in our healthcare system... it did not. When I asked him how many times he had performed this particular surgery, he said it was only a "handful" of times. Still unconvinced, I forged ahead with the surgery, feeling like I had no other option.

In the days following my surgery I was on a liquid diet, and slowly but surely, like you as a baby, I graduated to softer foods and more solids. My confidence grew with every bite and successful swallow, just as yours did, until I wasn't afraid to eat anymore. In the months that followed, I had no episodes and I was shocked at how this surgery had changed my life so completely.

A decade later, I still have episodes—you will, of course, have noticed them—moments where my face starts to strain, when my esophagus wants to take a break, the chest pains return, and I have to run to the bathroom, but thank goodness they are few and far between. I'm truly grateful to have been given what seems like a second chance to live my life the way that I have always wanted—on my terms, not dictated by this disorder.

I'm not telling you all of this for your pity (maybe for some extra hugs). I'm telling you this so that you can learn from my story. Learn how to deal with any hardships you will face, because you will face some; it's inevitable. Everyone deals with them in their own way, and while I may not be able to help you when the time comes, my hope is that you can take something from my struggles that will make it easier for you to deal with yours.

You come from a long line of women whose lives have not been easy. Maybe I'll tell you their stories one day. Many of them have been shamed into submission, not allowed to feel or talk about their suffering. This has only amplified the power that it had over their lives. For a long time, I felt that I, too, had to follow in their footsteps... that talking about hard things would only do more harm than good (and for a time, this was partly true).

It was certainly easier to do. For a while, every time that I wanted to try and talk about this, it was like reliving both the physical pain and emotional toll that it took on me. I couldn't talk about it without crying. But the truth of the matter is this: I was muting my own voice by not talking about the struggles I have gone through. I just wanted to move on and not let this illness define me, but that was exactly what I was doing by not talking about it. I was giving it the power to control what I said, how I said it, and to whom. So here I am writing about it and about what I have learned, no longer a captive being held against my will. While each person has their own lessons they take away from their struggles, here are just some of the things that I have learned from mine:

Eat the ice cream; take the trip; buy the shoes.

Once the fear of eating had dissipated, I had this new sense of freedom. My uncle told me, "eat whatever you want now; when you're older, doctors will prevent you from eating all the good stuff." I really took this to heart and you should, too. While it seemed like almost everyone my age was on a health kick, eating kale, avocado toast, and doing every diet you could imagine, I was running in the opposite direction. I wanted to catch up on all of the food that I had missed out on eating in the last decade. This was the age where my metabolism was probably going to be the best that it was ever going to be, so I had to take advantage!

I remember one night I was at a friend's house soon after my surgery and I managed to eat my first Haägen-Daz ice cream bar entirely without any issues. I couldn't even remember the last time I was able to eat ice cream without having an issue. My friend offered me a second one. I ate it no problem. She offered me a THIRD and in that moment I was truly on the mend (side note: friends that offer you three ice creams without any judgements are friends you should have for life). Now, I'm not saying to do this everyday, but food is not only meant to nourish you, but to be enjoyed, so eat whatever brings that joy. If you love kale, more power to you. If you feel like eating pancakes for dinner, don't think twice—eat the pancakes. Too many girls develop an unhealthy relationship with food because they worry about what everyone else does and they forget this simple fact.

At the same time, I also started to do the things I had always wanted to but let my illness prevent me from doing. There was certainly a lot to catch up on, and so one of the first things I did was take some time off work and went travelling around the globe. I bought my first apartment and moved out on my own for the first time. I started dating. I moved to Chicago, a city where I didn't know a single person, to work. I would have never even considered any of these things before because of my illness. I was too worried about what I would be able to eat, what would happen if I couldn't eat, and who would be able to support me if I was alone and struggling.

In summary, cram all that you can into this transitory life and go with your gut. If you want to eat ice cream, eat it. If you want to travel the world, do it. If you want to buy those nice shoes you've been eyeing, buy them. I will support you 100% (unless it's something that appears to threaten your safety, of course). In my experience, you regret very little when you go with your instinct.

Don't waste time going down the "Why Me?" wormhole.

Once the novelty of this new found "freedom" wore off, I began to really think about what I had gone through and the negative thoughts came rushing in. I began to think about what my life could have been like in the last decade had I not been sick. In this parallel universe, would I still have gone to the same university? Would I have the same career? Would I have been more outgoing? Would I be in a serious relationship? I also asked the universe *Why me? Why did this have to happen to me?* I was a good person. I followed the rules. I did everything that was asked of me. So why did this happen to me and not to someone else? I think a lot of people that go through hardship ask themselves this, and often it results in a crisis of faith (if you believe in God). At the beginning of my illness, I prayed a lot, hoping that if I prayed hard enough and long enough that perhaps I would be cured. But God doesn't work that way. Sometimes prayers aren't enough. Sometimes you have to go through these trials because it gets you to where you need to be. Unfortunately, you don't have the coles notes (am I dating myself by saying "coles notes"?) to your story and you don't know what He has planned for you in the end.

All of these questions that I was asking myself were alluding to the fact that I would have been better off or end up in a better place than I currently was. It was only until I met your dad and I had you that I stopped asking myself those questions. I realized that I was right where I was supposed to be. One of the reasons your dad and I connected in the first place was because of the fact that we both faced hardship in our early years. The ease and comfort I found in talking to him about what I had gone through was just what I needed, and I'm truly grateful to have him as a partner in this life. In any other alternate universe, I probably wouldn't have met your dad and had you, and who would want to live a life without you guys?

The truth is, you will never find answers to these questions, so asking them is futile. I probably asked them hoping to help make sense of what happened, hoping to find meaning in all of the pain. But there are things in life that you won't be able to explain. You've just got to come to terms with that. I went through something hard, as most people in their life do. It was painful but I was lucky enough to come out the other side relatively unscathed. Once I accepted this, I was able to let go of this cloud of negativity that was following me everywhere, and I was able to get on with living the life that I had always dreamed of.

Love the body you have, not the one you wish you had.

The human body is not made to last. It is something we all have to come to terms with. The bodies that we had in our early years that were more limber and able to heal themselves quicker slowly start to degrade. Aches and pains become more frequent and our bones become brittle and frail. As we age a simple bodily function that we once took for granted may become a monumental task. For me this realization came way too early in life. Something as simple as swallowing became an accomplishment for me if I could do it successfully without struggle. For the longest time I hated my body. I hated what it was doing to me. I hated the things that it had stopped me from doing, and I hated the person that it was making me become. But I have grown to love and accept it. You will likely find some sort of fault with your body as well. Just remember that while your body is not perfect, it's the only body you have and it's doing its best. Mine was able to provide you with a warm and loving home for nine months, so I think I'll forgive some of its shortcomings.

Listen to your body and stick up for it when it needs you to.

I hate doctors. I always have, and probably always will. You probably can appreciate why based on my experiences with them. I think most doctors don't go into their profession for the right reasons and don't treat their patients with the respect they deserve. Having said all of this, I don't want YOU to hate them. I've had a history of bad experiences over the past 15+ years that have led me to this conclusion and it has eroded any trust that I had in them, but there is still hope for you.

What I've learned is that you can't just rely on your doctors to figure it out; you bear some responsibility as well. Perhaps if I had been more persistent with my doctors over that span of time, or explained what I had been going through as I have now, we would have discovered my illness sooner. But at the time I was a child and I didn't know that I could speak up. Often there is this barrier that is created between doctor and patient that can make you feel like you can't voice your concerns, and that the doctor is always right. But I've seen in countless cases, not only my own, where this just isn't true. The doctor may not be right; they may not have all the information; they may not understand just how bad you feel or why it doesn't feel normal to you.

The best advocate for your health isn't your parents or your doctor; it's you. You know your body better than anyone else, and only you will know when something is off. Pay attention to your body and the signs that it's giving you. Most likely, if you notice a change, there is something wrong. If your doctor dismisses it, or the feeling persists, don't be afraid to speak louder until they listen—or find someone else who will. If you feel unsure about the doctor's recommendations, voice your concerns—don't just go along with it. Don't let ten years go by before you finally get answers, because it may be too late.

Even now, ten years after my surgery, I have to remind myself of the lessons that I learned from all of this. It's easy to get caught up in the day-to-day grind and to forget to listen to your body, not feed your soul, and to get lost in all the negativity in the world. But I am constantly reminded that Achalasia is incurable. It will stay with me forever and my symptoms may return even worse than before. Every time I look at myself in the mirror and see the scars on my belly from my surgery, they are a reminder that I have to make this time count. I want to be able to look back on my life and see both the struggles and the triumphs and be content with the life I've lived.

To be sure the years before my diagnosis were hard, they were painful, and I missed out on a lot, but it wasn't all terrible. There were still moments of laughter amongst all of the pain, and I have to hold onto those good moments as well. Why is it so easy for us to cling onto the difficult things and not the good, I wonder? I don't have all of the answers and this is something that I myself am still working on.

I have a rare illness; so rare, in fact, that I haven't actually met anyone else who has this disorder. For the longest time I felt like people wouldn't understand, so why bother talking about it? What I've come to realize is that everybody goes through tough times. Some may be able to hide it better than others, but it's part of life. There are ups and downs in everyone's life, not just ups. People may not be able to relate to the specifics, but at some basic human level we can all appreciate the toll that going through something difficult can take.

We need to rethink how hard things are dealt with and talked about. This idea that difficult or hard is bad and should be swept under the rug and forgotten about is just not true. Our hardships can be painful, crippling, and seem never-ending, but they aren't a reflection of who we are as people. Our hardships should not define us, but oftentimes we allow them to. I certainly did. The more I talk about it, the less power I let it have over me. I've come to realize that this illness is just a chapter in my life. It may want to be the leading lady in my biopic, but really it is only meant to play a cameo. Only I can dictate the path my life will take and the person I want to be—not my friends, not my family, and most certainly not this illness, and I am determined that my story will have a happy ending. It is my sincere hope that your story does, too.

Chapter 15
VICKI SPINDLOE

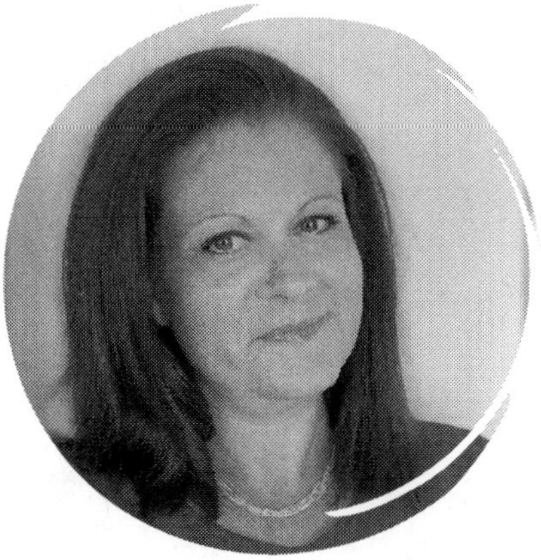

Instagram @leadwithkindness247

"When I grow up, I will marry my true love and live happily forever..."

In Grade 9, this tall skinny boy with braces came into my life and I fell head over heels for him. I knew that he was the one, and that we were going to be together forever and have this lasting love. My future was going to turn out just as I had always dreamed it would. My sweetheart and I met at a wedding, so for someone like me who believes that things happen for a reason, this girl knew that it was fate and this relationship was meant to be.

I grew up in your typical nuclear family with two parents and siblings. My parents' relationship was perfect (well, in my eyes) and they were amazing role models in showing us (my sisters and I) what a marriage and partnership should be like. I spent my entire childhood living in an environment that was happy. I witnessed that "happily ever after" kind of love/marriage... but now I know that your happily ever after does not always happen the first-time around!

Hi. My name is Vicki. I'm a registered early childhood educator and owner/creator of Lead with Kindness, a mother to two amazing children, and a wife to a wonderful, hard working man who I call my "Knight in a Hooters Hat." I will expand more on that a little bit later, but he is the light at the end of a very dark tunnel, the one who helped repair a shattered life and allowed me to slowly take down the wall around my broken heart (a wall that I never imagined I would need). Sometimes life can throw you a hard right hook, but you can handle hard stuff—and don't forget that!

'Til Death Do Us Part

Remember that tall skinny boy I met at a wedding and fell in love with the moment I saw him across the room...?

Just after our 8-year dating anniversary on a cold and rainy Sunday afternoon while sitting in my parents' living room, he pulled out that little black box and popped the question: "Will you spend the rest of your life with me?" Of course I cried and said YES!!!

My fairytale story was about to begin...

On July 7, 2007...7.7.7, which is supposedly a super lucky day, I had my fairytale wedding that every little girl dreams of. We were the first couple from our group of friends to get married, and I will be honest in saying that at times it put a bit of a strain on our marriage. I was wanting that newly married couple life, but my hubby was still living life like he was single. I wanted the date nights or weekends away with just my husband, and he was making plans with the boys or heading away with the gang for another night of drinking and partying. At times it felt like his friends took more of a priority over me, and that was difficult for me to understand. I always wondered why and would ask myself why he even married me. Things became even more challenging when we decided to start a family.

Soon to Be Three

Only a year into my newly wedded life I found out that we were expecting, but our relationship was put to the test when we experienced our first loss. I grieved the loss of our pregnancy alone, and he grieved by going to a house party. Normally I am the type of person who tends to hide my feelings, and this time was no different. In his defense, he did ask if it was okay if he went out and I did reassure him that it was alright with me. I guess I just did not want to waste any more energy fighting with him; I was exhausted already.

When a person is at a breaking point with their emotions, however, one can certainly discover a lot about themselves and how strong they can be in handling tough stuff. This was just the beginning for me on how to find the strength to keep pushing through. I had no clue at the time how much I would need to lean on that strength and how much it would be tested repeatedly.

You see, no one ever plans on having to deal with hard things in life, but we all do. No one wakes up with the thought of, "what heartache or traumatic event is going to happen today?" I know that I never started my day saying, "today is the day I will have a miscarriage."

I had never imagined that I would struggle with infertility, but after we experienced losses over and over, I felt like it would never happen. It put a huge strain and even more tension on our already very rocky relationship. At the time, I wanted a baby more to hopefully keep my husband at home, rather than him always wanting to be with his friends. I peed on that stick and prayed it was for the last time. We waited 12 weeks to find out that our little bundle of joy was still inside and thriving. It became clear that my husband wanted this next chapter just as much as I did. We were finally going to be PARENTS!!!

We could not hold in the excitement and happiness and began counting down to the day that we would welcome this bundle of joy into the world. Finally, our marriage and life were heading in the right direction and things were falling into place. We were happy!

Well, that is what I thought...

There I was, eight months pregnant, sitting across the kitchen table staring at my husband. I could see his mouth moving, but I could not hear the words. Time stood still—frozen in the moment—that moment when my world, my life, and my dreams just shattered.

Frozen in That Moment

> ***"This is a bad dream that I cannot wake up from. This cannot be real!"***

I sat there frozen, staring at him, replaying the words repeatedly. As the words left his mouth, all I could do was put my hands on my belly—the belly where our little guy was growing, the little guy that was about to enter the world in just a few weeks—and that is all that I could focus on right in that moment. My husband's words seemed to keep repeating in my head, or maybe my husband was just repeating himself, yet my mind couldn't focus on anything at that moment. I was frozen in that moment.

You are probably asking yourself, "What words? What did he say?" Well, I truly never imagined that this would ever happen to me, but there I was. I knew that whatever happened next, I was going to have to work hard to get through it. You know, pull up your big girl pants, as they say. I had to snap back to reality, as this was as real as it gets. I was about to come face-to-face with a really hard situation, but I knew that no matter what, I was going to get through it.

It was around 11:00 p.m. on a cold and snowy December night when I received a call from my husband. His father had recently had heart surgery, so my husband had been staying a few nights at his house when he was needed. So, when my husband asked me if I would drive to his dad's house during a snowstorm (and eight months preggo), I really did not think anything of it, nor did I see that the second worst thing in my life was about to go down (the first was the passing of my dad... that is a whole other hard to handle situation in my life.)

I walked into the house like I had done a million times before, and found my husband sitting at the kitchen table, but the look on his face had me concerned. He looked scared; he looked terrified, and he could not even look at me. He sat with his head down, and completely silent.

Then the words began to flow, and my heart began to shatter...

"I have been seeing someone else."... "I have feelings for her."... "I am sorry."

The more he said, the more time froze. The more he talked,

the more my heart shattered. The more he tried to explain, the more my world started spinning out of control—and the more my fairytale life disappeared.

Things went silent, and now it was my turn. With my hand firmly on my belly, feeling my little guy kick and roll, I began to put my thoughts into words, and then time thawed; I was no longer frozen.. I will be honest; as much as I wanted to be super strong and not show any emotion, that just was not possible, because how does a pregnant woman keep her hormones in control after hearing that her husband was having an affair?! At that very moment, life just felt like it had ended.

Where does one even begin with finding out more information, or putting all of this info into perspective? I started with "Who is she?" "Do I know her?" "When did it start?" And the questions just kept coming.

The answers that I was receiving, made me once again frozen in the moment. The moment he replied "Yes, you know her," followed by her name... I felt sick, like physically ill. It made me want to throw up (and not because of the all-day morning sickness) to think about her and to think that only a few weeks prior to this moment, she had been sleeping with my hubby while at the same time planning my baby shower (yes, she was a friend). How does one even do something like that? What honestly goes through your head when you look at someone the day after you have been in bed with her husband? One thing I knew was that my fairytale life with him was over.

The minutes, hours, days, and weeks after his confession all seemed to blend together. As the pieces to this puzzle began to unfold, I was faced with the tough decision about how to move forward and figure out the next steps. Life just seemed to be a blur as I walked through this. I started to take the steps to process all of the things running through my mind, but overthinking and overanalyzing took me down a path of destruction—and the blame and the shame started. The big question on my mind each day was *how am I going to bring this bundle of joy into the world...alone?!*

Stronger than the Shame

> ***"If only I was a better person, this wouldn't have happened."***
>
> ***"I don't deserve to be loved."***

I began to blame myself, began the negative self-talk, and started to put myself down. My personality has always been bright, uplifting, and with a positive attitude, but that light inside was dark and dim. I felt like another version of myself was growing inside. I began to feel like this happened *to* me, but now I know that it all happened *for* me. The person I was back then was broken. I could not see that life was putting me into this situation because it was meant for me to believe more in myself, and to know that I was a badass bitch who was capable of anything.

When I looked in the mirror the following days, it was extremely hard to see anything positive. I saw a woman who should have been better at making her husband happy. I saw a woman who drove her husband into the arms of another woman. I saw a woman who should have done things differently. I saw all of the negative in myself and questioned who I was as a person. I blamed myself for what my husband had done. It had to be something I did, or maybe it was because of something I didn't do.

But in all reality, I had absolutely nothing to do with these two grown-ass adults making the choice that they did, because in all honesty, they had many other choices and still chose to sneak around for months. What angered me the most was when the bitch had the audacity to reach out to me because she wanted to explain her side. Here we are, ten years later, and I still have never spoken a single word to her. Nothing can be said to change what happened or even how I feel about it. Her side means nothing to me.

Once the strong, confident version of myself came to the realization that I was no longer allowing the blame to be put on me, it allowed the feelings to be replaced with anger—a level of anger that I have never felt before. I was incredibly angry at both of them, but if I am honest, I was angrier at his mistress than I was at my husband. Like, sure, he could have told her stories like "my wife and I are splitting up" or "I am leaving my wife for you," but she knew; she saw that we were still together and that we were creating a family together. We were planning the next chapter with each other. I always thought... *What if he had an affair with someone I didn't know?* Would I have felt differently? Maybe I would not have gone completely bat shit crazy thinking about the past and all of the times that I remember them being together.

Cue the feelings of shame and embarrassment. How did I not see any of the signs leading up to this? How could I have been so blind? There had to have been signs! Once more information began to surface, however, the signs and events leading up to it all became much clearer. I was embarrassed that I never saw this coming and wondered how many people knew but never said anything. I just wanted to hide away from the world.

I was completely ashamed and afraid of what other people thought. Were they judging me and blaming me? Did they also think that I had caused this? This was certainly something that was hard for me to deal with, and it made my social anxiety worse. I have an amazing support system, but at the time I lied to everyone close to me about where my husband was after we split. After a few months had passed, my immediate family probably had concerns, but no one said anything. They were more excited because my due date arrived.

I could not tell them. I needed things to remain the same. For now, I needed this affair—this heartache, this life changing moment—to remain hidden from them. I needed to do this one last thing and have faith that it was going to be as magical as I had been dreaming of for nine months.

Life was about to head down the next unknown road, and I would be doing it alone!

Just You & Me, Kid

The day had finally arrived! My water broke, and I went into labour. Parts of that day went as planned and other moments felt awkward and emotionally hard to handle. The last thing that I wanted to do was go through this joyful experience with my soon to be EX-husband, but here I was breathing through contractions listening to him tell me how great I was doing. Even though I wished I had never called him or that he would just leave, I would also never have taken this moment of seeing his son being born away from him. That is how I know I am a good, kind person. This is when I knew that the road I was about to travel along, was something that I could handle...like a boss!!! Was it going to be easy? Nope, not even close.

My family gathered and met my little guy, and there was only pure joy, happiness, and love in that room. You see, this positive energy in the environment was created because my family had no clue about what had been going down the last few weeks behind the scenes (except my middle sister). It was extremely tough to keep this from my family, but I knew that I wasn't going to enter the wonderful stage of motherhood with anger and hate in the room. You see, the last thing I wanted was to think back and remember how toxic my delivery was, or how toxic people were to each other. Instead, I look back and recall the smiles, laughter, and pure love that happened in that room that very cold January night.

I did this for my little guy. I did this so that when I show him photos of the night that he came into our lives, he will see the happiness shared amongst everyone. I do have a photo with a family friend who knew the dirty little secret, and you can see the hate in her face as she sat beside my ex holding our little guy. It is just another painful reminder of the hurt an affair can cause, and let's be real: no one wants to continue to relive that shit every time you look back on past photos.

As happy and joyful as that night was, however, it was also unbearable to continue to keep up with a fake smile. I don't know how fake people do it all the time, because that shit is exhausting. I was truly relieved when the nurse said visiting hours were over, but this was when my ex-husband realized this new mama was faking kindness—and where I knew I had the power and the strength to take control. I remember the shocked look on his face when the words "You can leave now, we don't need you" left my mouth. After 14 hours, I could finally breathe. I had a plan for the next few months, but I sat there crying because the future was unclear.

It was super late; I believe around 2:00 a.m. or so. I remember holding him and looking at him. I kissed him on the forehead and said, "Well, buddy, it's just you and me now. I promise to always put you first and I will protect you and keep you safe."

It was time for this new mama to put on her big girl pants and dig deep inside to find the strength to tackle life, because it was not going to be an easy road from here on out. Single mom life, here I come!

I did have a small moment of postpartum depression, but it thankfully was noticed and dealt with quickly. I had it mostly because I was angry and jealous that my ex could do normal things, like just get up and go anywhere—you know, live that bachelor life, with no responsibility—but here I was, living as a single mom with a newborn. I didn't ask for this life. I didn't sign up for this life, and I wanted it to end. There, however, was a strong inner voice that said *nope,* my ex-husband is not going to take this from me. He is not going to walk away all happy and carefree, and I am going to show him that he gave up the best things in life.

After a few months of motherhood, I had a long conversation with that scared, depressed, afraid, anxious woman in the mirror. I told her that enough was enough. It was time to put this baby boy first and do what is best for him. I deserved these firsts as a new mom and deserved to live a happy life. Here is what I have learned so far with all of this: things happen for a reason, and this situation happened for me to realize that I am capable of being a strong single mama. I did not need to depend on anyone else. I can create my own happiness in life.

Not only was the first year of motherhood tough, but I also added dating into the mix. I had not been on a date in over 14 years, and now I was going to put myself on the dating scene as a single mom (with an infant), dealing with a separation. Let's be real for a second: I did work really hard at getting my body back (maybe even better) to how it was before having my son. I think they call it the "revenge body." However, I was scared to death to put myself out there, and where does one even start?

I was afraid to find someone who was just going to break my heart, so that is when I built this protective wall. I dated a few, I had fun with some more, but I never had a real connection and began to think that I would never find the right guy. It was hard to make plans to go out, especially when I had a baby at home to take care of. At the time, my ex was only having our little guy for day visits, so any dates I did go on were planned around that time. Also, I didn't want anyone to meet my little guy until I knew 100% that it was going to last, as I didn't want my son to make connections with people and then have them leave (I know he would never know since he was an infant). I did have thoughts of just dating all of my ex's single friends—you know, like rub it in his face—but that did not feel right, and I would probably eventually have to hang out with my ex and that thing he was dating (the mistress). I made sure that my ex knew that I was dating and having all of the fun.

Many of the people I dated were definitely on different paths in life than me. I was a single mom, and they were living the bachelor life. I was responsible for keeping a tiny human alive and most of the guys were just responsible for themselves. Also, I was a parent and many of the guys couldn't or were not ready to step into the step-parent role. I thought that maybe it would just be my little guy and me forever...there is more to life than dating. It was time to face the fact that I would grow old alone.

I once again started to play the negative thoughts game. Maybe I am not good enough, or pretty enough, or I don't deserve to find love... *bitch, please—you are an amazing person who is just currently trying to navigate the shitty hand you were dealt*. Things happen for a reason, and this was just another hurdle in the game of life that I had to get through.

One day that all changed when I went to a friend's house party (which I wasn't originally going to attend) and the host of the party randomly introduced me to this guy...a random guy in a Hooters hat. He was certainly not the type of guy I had been dating, but there was just something about him and I knew that I needed to get to know him more. I was very cautious heading into this relationship, but he was one person who knew my ex but wasn't in that group of friends. He also knew I had a son but respected that my little guy came first, and he was so understanding when plans had to change at the last second. He understood my situation because he had had the same kind of relationship breakup. He was the one date I kept secret, because I didn't want my ex to ruin it (he tried a few times). Fast forward 11 years, and that guy has shown me what true love is and has made it clear that people can have a fairytale ending. It might not be all sunshine and rainbows, but I know that together we can get through the tough things in life. Just know that things happen for you. Embrace the positive in every situation and eventually the clouds will clear.

Learning As We Go

The first year was such a joyful time as I watched my little guy grow and hit all of those big milestones, but there was also this side of me that surfaced—and it was out of character for me. It was the spiteful side; the side that wanted to rub it in my ex's face that I got to witness all of our son's first milestones, and he did not. Deep down I loved that I shared these moments with my partner and my ex's partner missed out. You know, I was always the type of person to play fairly, but I wanted this all to myself and I wanted to come out the winner.

Realistically, however, that is not how parenting works. It is hard to share even as an adult, and it becomes even harder when you are sharing a child with someone and you're still kind of hating that person. It ate away at me every time my son left for his dad's house, and it wasn't even because he was with his dad, but more so that he was with the girl who took this family life from us. I knew that no matter how I felt about her or what anger still lingered, I had to "be the bigger person," as they say, because in the end, my son deserved to have a relationship with his father. So, every other weekend, I put on those big girl pants.

As hard as it may be sometimes, I must put my feelings aside, because it's important to see the situation from the other person's point of view. I would never want to be in my ex's shoes watching my son grow up from the sidelines (or every other weekend), so here is where I had to find those big girl pants again and wear them with such strength, and realize that the next hard thing was about to come my way... co-parenting!

Co-Parenting Challenges

> ***"Ok, Vic, so when it comes to L, we will make all the decisions together..." says the ex.***

Well, here is where co-parenting is sometimes exceedingly difficult and can feel like you are running in circles. Who does he think he is telling me what we are going to do, and how it is going to be? He lost that right when he had an affair and left us.

At the beginning this was hard for me to deal with because I wanted all of the control and I wanted to keep my little guy with me 24/7, but that is not what was best in the long run. Here's the thing: from the day our divorce papers were signed, it has been me in the driver's seat and who controlled how this was all going to play out. It was going to be my way or no way. I wanted to say when and where and how. At first, it worked because my son was an infant, so for obvious reasons our son needed to be with me more, but we worked out a schedule that would be in our son's best interest. There was going to come a time when I knew I did not want my son to look back and blame me for not allowing him to have a relationship with his dad from the start—and thus began our co-parenting relationship.

Over the years it has been challenging, yet rewarding all at the same time. The hardest part of letting my son go is not having the ability to control what he does. I 100% trust my ex when it comes to doing what is best and keeping our son safe, but not being in control of what my son does there really bugs me. It is also hard to not want to buy things so that the child picks you over the other parent. I have had to have some tough talks with my ex, because that is no way to raise a child together. Another difficult part of co-parenting is splitting up the holidays, which is even harder to deal with when the other parent is not really into traditions. Over the years I have learnt to go over the top and be a little more "extra," as they say, when it is my turn to have our son for a holiday.

Our journey of co-parenting is still in progress, and I am sure that there will be more hurdles to jump. One hurdle that I know is in our future is the day that our son asks why we are not together and wants to know what happened. How does one explain this to a child?

I was not the villain in my marriage, and I will be damned if I am going to end up being the villain in my son's story. No matter what hurdles his father and I must face in the future, my little guy will always come first, and I will do what is best for him.

Over the years I have learnt a lot about myself—not only as a mom, but also as an ex-wife. I am still working through all of the feelings that arise at times, but I continue to grow from them.

leadher
PUBLISHING

For more information about LeadHer Publishing books, author projects, and resources, visit *leadherpublishing.com*

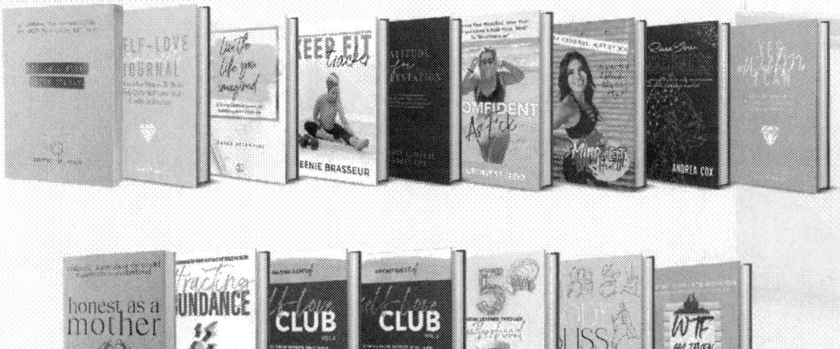

Manufactured by Amazon.ca
Bolton, ON

26609020R00129